PELICAN BOOKS

YOGA

Ernest Wood, born in 1883 in Manchester, took an early interest in science and philosophy, and received his advanced education at the Manchester College of Technology, gaining Firsts in Physics, Chemistry, and Geology. As a young man he went to India and took up in 1910 the post of Headmaster of a Congress High School, preparing students for the University of Madras. After that he became managing secretary of a group of thirty-seven schools and colleges, and was also Principal and President of the Sind National College and the Madanapalle College, of the Universities of Bombay and Madras. All along he was deeply interested in the Yoga and Vedanta philosophies of India, and learned to read them in the original Sanskrit language, while associating closely with scholars and yogis. During his long residence in India Professor Wood wrote many books on education, psychology, and Indian philosophy, besides making a number of translations. He was President and Dean of the American Academy of Asian Studies, a graduate school in San Francisco. He died in 1965.

ERNEST WOOD

YOGA

PENGUIN BOOKS

Penguin Books Ltd, Harmondsworth, Middlesex, England
Penguin Books, 625 Madison Avenue, New York, New York 10022, U.S.A.
Penguin Books Australia Ltd, Ringwood, Victoria, Australia
Penguin Books Canada Ltd, 41 Steelcase Road West, Markham, Ontario, Canada
Penguin Books (N.Z.) Ltd, 182–190 Wairau Road, Auckland 10, New Zealand

—

First published 1959
Reprinted 1961
Reprinted with revisions 1962
Reprinted 1964, 1965, 1967, 1968, 1970, 1971, 1972, 1973, 1974, 1975, 1976, 1977

—

Copyright © the Estate of Ernest Wood, 1959, 1962

—

Made and printed in Great Britain
by Hazell Watson & Viney Ltd,
Aylesbury, Bucks
Set in Monotype Baskerville

CONTENTS

PRONUNCIATION OF SANSKRIT WORDS

Vowels: a as in India or England or America.

             ā as in father.

             i as in kin.

             ī as in machine.

             u as in put.

             ū as in pool.

             e as in grey.

             o as in home.

             ai as in aisle, or as i in isle.

             au as ow in how.

Consonants: k, g, ch, j, t, d, p, n, m, y, r, l, v, sh, s, h – as in English. th, ph, etc., are all sounded with h unblended as in hot-house, haphazard, etc.

             The combination jn presents the only difficulty, being sounded slightly differently in different provinces. The reader will be safe in giving it somewhat the sound of gny as in French words such as compagne and compagnon.

Type: Sanskrit words are given in italics, with the long vowels marked, as *ā*, *ī*, and *ū*. Some Sanskrit words, however, have been adopted into English; these are printed in ordinary type and the long vowels are not usually marked, except in the first instance, where it is given to ensure correct pronunciation. Such are yoga, yogi, nirvana, karma, etc.

INTRODUCTION

In this presentation of yogic thought and practice I have endeavoured to maintain the entire background of classical literature on the subject. Therefore the reader will find a sprinkling of Sanskrit words, which are original terms of specific and technical value. These words, however, are presented mostly in brackets, so that they may be ignored by the general reader without any loss to his complete understanding of the subject. Their presence in the brackets will show the Sanskrit scholar and specialist exactly what is being referred to in the English rendering in each case. For the reader who wishes to understand these words as the basis of a vocabulary of yoga for future classical study we have provided a glossary, to which he can easily refer until they have become familiar.

Our reason for maintaining the classical background should be clear. There were in the old days in India strata of society which provided for men and families dedicated to religion and philosophy, and thus able to study and practise these without such distractions as we have in modern living. These groups gave themselves to this study in a definitely scientific and factual manner, with application in practice and pragmatic consideration of results. Yoga thus grew up as applied religion, and at the same time the science of introspectional psychology – introspectional meaning not retreat from factual experience, but direct inspection of the contents of the mind, yet not ignoring the application of the knowledge so gained to the body and the environment.

I have endeavoured to cover practically the entire range of classical literature on the subject, which is by no means a dead literature but mainly a collection of textbooks which are fully in use and highly regarded by the present-day yogis in India – whether those who give their full time to the subject, or those exceedingly numerous persons in all walks of life who set aside a little special time for it every day and allow its motives and its gains to permeate the rest of their time. While thus presenting the subject in the classical manner, I have also consciously and unconsciously woven into it my great familiarity over decades with those who actually practise yoga and regard it as the most important part of their lives, both in personal practice and in social application. I have also related it to modern psychological knowledge.

INTRODUCTION

Bringing the material of so many classical texts together in the present book, I have thought it best to group the material according to practical usefulness, as will be seen by a perusal of the chapter titles. This I have thought preferable to the method of presenting résumés and explanations of particular texts in separate chapters, which would give the reader the labour of much cross-reference for the acquisition of clear and mature ideas on specific points.

In treating the subject-matter I have endeavoured to give just and equal attention to every part of it. The reader will therefore find, I hope, adequate treatment of the highest goals, the awakening of the higher mind, the self realization of the human spirit, the discovery of God, as well as of bodily and mental health, and the benefits which yoga brings into daily life – given time and ripening – both in mind and heart and in circumstances. The whole shows that the law of good is as potent in material gains as in the enrichment and strengthening of the inner life.

It is shown, I think, that yoga is in every way integral living, including the whole man – material, mental, ethical, spiritual – by which each of the levels of our being serves all the others and results in complete sanity and happiness.

It has been asked whether in yoga there is something for everybody. The answer is 'yes'. One standard work on the subject, written over a thousand years ago, states: 'It is for children, adults and the aged, for the well and the ill, for the poor and the rich.' There is one condition, however – the individual has to do the work himself. Life, after all, rests only in the individual. As Emerson put it in one of his poems:

> The cordial quality of pear or plum
> Rises as gladly in the single tree
> As in whole orchards resonant with bees.

Yoga is something to do, yet its benefits are not something to make, but something to take. Its teachers follow the method of the gardener, who provides soil, water, and sunshine, allowing the plant its own power of life, not the methods of the builders and the sculptors, who add or chip away. Our modern scientists now know that the age of natural selection is gone, and men must look to themselves, not their material environment, for the direction and impulse needed for their future progress.

ERNEST WOOD

CHAPTER I

THE WHY AND THE HOW OF YOGA

WHY do so many Hindus 'take to yoga'? The chief reason is that from childhood they have heard about it, and have been familiar with legendary stories of great sages and saints and heroes of the past who have shown serenity and ability and strength – all gained through yoga – altogether superior to the lot of the masses of the people among whom they find that they have been born. They have perhaps listened to some of the numerous lectures on the subject or have read some of the books. Above all, many have looked into the famous yoga teachings of Patanjali, written down in his *Yoga Sūtras* more than three hundred years B.C.

Those yoga *sūtras* (aphorisms) affirm at the outset that human unhappiness results from man's acceptance of a state of servitude to the low condition of his own mind.

They do not leave it at that, however, but they show how men can overcome this condition, and in time become like the sages and saints and heroes of their dreams, and, further, that they can also pass on into spiritual worlds – no less real than this – in which they will be veritable masters of life, or, in brief, that they can win competency for citizenship in the Kingdom of God.

Their belief does not set the future and the present at odds with each other. In their eyes the same mode of life that leads to what we may call the Kingdom – the word, however, is Independence (*kaivalya*) – also leads to the greatest happiness and the most felicitous conditions of existence on earth. Health, beauty, peace, prosperity, and every reasonable felicity result from the same ethics, mental disciplines, and type of endeavour as lead to a future free from the restrictions of earthly life.

Or, if the candidate for happiness through yoga chooses to do so, he can postpone his ultimate aims and think only of a series of future lives on earth with a conspicuous decrease of its objectionable features and increase of desirable ones, by the same effective and agreeable methods.

The candidate can proceed step by step, keeping his eye on the ground and doing one thing after another, or he can choose an ideal or an ideal person or mahātmā as his goal, and approach a teacher or *guru* for guidance towards it. The legends are full of noble examples, and the *gurus* have been many even within historical times. The *guru* is one who has experienced divine freedom in his consciousness, and knows the means by which it may be attained.

In some Western writings this state of freedom or independence has been called 'cosmic consciousness'. If this is to fit the yogic conception we must not use the word cosmic as meaning all-inclusive, but only – if one may say only – the direct perception and experience of the divine consciousness which is free from the troubles already mentioned, and is also inherently joyful.

Perhaps the first thing that the candidate learns is that his future does not depend upon fortunate material circumstances. There must however be enough. This could be expressed, and is expressed, in some of the books, in the following terms: 'Be glad that you are a man, and now do not be so foolish as to miss the opportunity this gives.'

It is for this purpose that the yogi attends to his bodily needs and welfare. Suicide would certainly lead nowhere. And neglect of the body will do no good. Still, the reasonable middle way is best. The candidate will learn that bodily greatness in the shape of uncommon muscular strength or skill in athletics will not help at all. The motto with reference to bodily strength may be said to be 'Enough is enough', but definitely also 'Enough is necessary'.

It may be thought by the enquirer or the novice that though a powerful body is not necessary for yoga a powerful mind is necessary – mind being defined as the totality of the functions of thinking, feeling, and willing. This too the student soon finds not to be the case. Once more 'Enough is enough', and once more 'Enough is necessary'. Great mental ability and special mental talent or genius are not required. On the other hand, stupidity, confusion, and dissipation can avert or destroy the 'enough'.

What of the non-aspirants to yoga? In India, a land where the idea of yoga is familiar to the least educated, and in which there is hardly anybody who has not seen a yogi[1], what is the state of the average person, who is not seeking yoga? These numerous persons are most surprisingly free from any anxiety or self-reproach in the matter. They take themselves quite peacefully. They say: 'I am not ready for yoga yet; I do not really want it now.' It never occurs to them to think 'I ought to want it'. They do not feel that there is any occasion for self-discontent or self-reproach. They take themselves as they find themselves, and say 'I am fond of the pleasures of eating and talking and sex' – mild as these may be in most cases in India. Oh, yes, they do have the idea that some day they will 'become perfect'. But it is not for now, and thus there is no internal conflict in their minds between the ideal and the actual, which creates such havoc in Western minds. One has indeed sometimes to warn the Western novice not to make of yoga another craving.

They also have no theory of 'now or never' to trouble them, for the belief acquired in childhood, seeming as natural as the mother-tongue and the ways of village life, is that the infinite future will offer them all the opportunity they need whenever they feel ready for it. They lose nothing by postponement. On all these accounts they are not ridden by anxiety. There are 'future lives'.

Aspirants to yoga are definitely classed in three divisions – beginners or those 'desiring to mount', those who have adopted some of the outlooks and practices of yoga, and the risen or 'mounted' ones (*yogārūdhas*). The word used for the mounted ones (*ārūdha*) is the same as that used to describe a person mounted on a horse. Such persons are well established in yogic science and skills, and can maintain their yoga practice in the midst of many distractions which would be upsetting to the novice. The beginners are those in whom

1. Pronounced yogee.

13

the desire to mount has somewhat arisen. It is like the 'awakening' of the Christian mystic, an awakening to the value, not merely to the understanding, but to the enjoyment of the yogic life. The clear-sighted and level-headed, even if simple, Indian, would not touch it were not the enjoyment factor there. If the thought were that there is to be enjoyment only at the end of the path of yoga, and not on the way, the candidate would expect to have a hard time before him. Undertaking the uncongenial, he would miss its value, and fall again and again. But if each part of it as he goes along becomes a pleasure, there will be progress indeed. Happiness and progress go hand in hand, with happiness leading. Pain has its use as an indicator of missing the way, and gives direction back into the path of happiness.

The aspirant suddenly, or dawningly, as the case may be, becomes alerted to that which he has seen but has not valued before, and this awakening, when it comes, will be natural, just as when the time arrives, in adolescence, it is natural for the young man or woman to find a new value in the company of the childhood playmate.

This awakening is also placed at the beginning of the yogic way by the philosophers of India when they speak of *viveka*, usually translated as discrimination, or discernment, as the very first step on the yogic path. It is often called the discovery of the inner man, because every one who makes the discovery identifies himself with the inner rather than with the outer. All people naturally identify themselves with the thinker rather than with the object of thought. It would be strange, would it not, if somebody seeing a camel thought he was a camel being seen by something else?

Patanjali opens his subject by pointing out that control of the vagrant impulses in the mind is the first necessary step. The mind grew up to serve the body – to help to fulfil desires, then to decide which desires to help or serve, then to work for the improvement of the desires, and at last to respond to the inner purpose of life and bring it more and more into effect. In the last case it learns a new obedience, well stated as 'Be still and know that I am God'. When there is not this obedience, the mind, taking up more and more responses to the conflicting demands of bodily pleasure and of pride, becomes a danger to itself.

In these days, in which it is well known that our civilized countries are reeking with cases of psychosomatic disorder, the follower of yoga might well say: 'I told you so. It is dangerous to have a mind in the condition in which most minds are kept. We tell you that you should do something about it before the real trouble begins. Besides, the same mind that pulls you down can also lift you up. It is not you yourself, but a subtle machine which must either obey your will or obey the behests of bodily pleasure or of pride.'

'What then should we do?' quavers the rather terrified enquirer. In response, Patanjali says, 'You must control the flow of ideas in your mind. If you will you can be your own true man, but if not you will be the pitiful victim of circumstances.'

And then Patanjali gives his first item of almost psychiatric psychology. He says:

The ideas are of five kinds, painful and pleasant. Right knowledge, wrong knowledge, fancy, sleep, and memories.[1]

This is greatly interesting. It means that every idea that rises before the mind is normally pigeon-holed into one of these five classes, quite automatically. Such is the almost unnoticed first operation it does – a healthy action. But look at the immediate implication of this proposition: if it should chance that an idea be wrongly ticketed, if a dream or a fancy is mistaken for reality, or if a memory is taken as a present fact – then there is aberration, and, if continued, insanity. A simple statement, indeed, of the cause of all our woes. Here is the root of our trouble; first of all, the mistaking of wrong knowledge for right knowledge, by regarding the non-eternal, impure, painful, and foreign constituents of body and mind as the Self, which in reality is eternal, pure, and happy.[2]

This error is the first of the five Sources of Trouble, which

1. *Yoga Sūtras*, i, 6.   2. *ibid.*, ii, 5.

is soon followed by egotistic, pleasure-seeking, pain-avoiding possessiveness.[1] Each of these five and all their progeny must be examined, and seen as what they are.

The candidate will have to practise thinking and not allow the emotions arising in prior ignorance about things to control the current of his thoughts. Neither past habits and prejudices, nor current excitement must be allowed to govern his mind.[2]

Although even the novice is well aware that circumstances can neither help nor hinder his endeavours (given the 'enough' already mentioned) he is also conscious that in his immature state of mind he is constantly being tempted back over the line separating him from those who are 'not ready' and 'do not want' yoga because they want the pleasures before mentioned. Such beginners are in transition between the two states, and are being pulled in two ways. They are perhaps excited sexually when they see a beautiful woman and they cannot resist that second, or even third, helping of tasty food, or that glass of wine, although they know that it will take the keen edge off their meditations and discrimination. For the time being they want pleasures of the senses (that is, of the world) more than they want self-perfection or God. On these occasions the enjoyments of the yogic path may be obscured by an excess of the less mature enjoyments of the body.

In such circumstances no one can find fault with them for resorting to discipline – first, by avoiding the tempting sights; secondly, by deliberately turning their thoughts back to their purpose, even sometimes with the aid of the muttered repetition of the names of God, or the name of their chosen ideal man or *guru* (teacher) should they happen to know one, or to know enough about one.

They are well aware that there is no such thing as 'naturalness' in these matters as far as humanity is concerned. This human mind has been too long in its present ways to leave human beings any natural instincts in sensuous matters, such as most of the animals have. The power-

1. *ibid.*, ii, 3.   2. *ibid.*, i, 12.

ful, intense, and concentrated searchlight of the human imagination opens its eyes as soon as the senses bring into the mind the picture of a pleasure-giving object. On the instant it sets that mind to work to obtain the object, or, failing that, to indulge in the sensation imaginatively. This can on no account be considered as natural, even though it may be the result of hereditary impulses.

With the simpler animals the bodily appetites are mostly geared to healthful activities and functions, as in the case of a huge and handsome lion seen at the zoo. There it sat with a big piece of raw meat between its paws, taking no notice of that appetizing food, but looking sleepily at the passers-by. That lion had been fed by a keeper a few minutes earlier, but before that had been pacing its cage and roaring ravenously when it heard the sounds of the man's approach, probably scenting the meat; but now it had satisfied its natural appetite with perhaps half of the supply, and would not be interested in the half still lying there until its needs (not memory of the pleasure of eating) once more excited its natural appetite.

It is worth while at this point to observe the distinction between the process of recognition and that of memory, as this will enforce our realization that control of mind, which is an essential and central feature of yoga practice, is necessary for health, whether of body or mind, and for the reaching to what may be beyond.

The psychology of the situation, which plays a large part in yoga practice, is that recognition is an earlier development than memory. Bodily pleasures and pains precede mentality. Then comes perception of the pain or pleasure-giving object, then recognition, then memory in which the picture of the object may arise even in its absence, then planning. It is the stream of memories and plannings that the would-be yogi finds it necessary to control.

The strong human memory prompts thoughts and imaginings even in the entire absence of a stimulating object. Indeed, the novice in yoga must introspectively observe what it is that he thinks about in his passive or restful moments, when no demands are being made upon him either bodily or mentally. What he finds there may be of this unnatural character, in which case some mental discipline may be very much in order. Regarding this the teacher Patanjali says:

When there is annoyance by bad thoughts, let there be reflection against them. This reflection to the contrary is: 'The bad thought of injury, untruth, theft, incontinence, or greed, whether done, caused to be done, or approved, whether preceded by greed, anger, or infatuation, whether mild, medium, or strong, results in endless pain and error.'[1]

This is mental discipline, and then:

From the habitual mood of friendliness, sympathy, gladness, and disregard respectively towards those who are happy, suffering, good and bad, comes purity of mind.[2]

Often and often the goal of the yogi is described in yoga literature as 'liberation'. The word is '*moksha*', and a better translation of it would be 'liberty'. This does not mean that the yogi is aiming at escape. Escape-from-it-all would be unconsciousness, which he does not expect. Escape from the disagreeables would leave him where he was before with regard to the agreeables, and no nearer to perfection nor divine experience. For the yogi, God is depicted as that being who is free, or, as the *Yoga Sūtras* have it, 'unaffected by troubles, works, and effects.'[3] Indeed when the yogi is given the option of practising devotion to God as one of the means to reaching the heights of contemplation, the idea is that in thinking of the divine he is picturing a being essentially free, and so he is looking forward to what he himself will become – free.

It is not that God is thought of as *having* or possessing freedom, but as *being* impregnably free. Little by little, or perhaps with a sudden insight, the yogi doing this, and having in his meditations – which are rational – eliminated from his idea or picture of himself everything inconsistent with

1. *ibid.*, ii, 33–4.   2. *ibid.*, i, 33.   3. *ibid.*, i, 24.

that freedom, will find that he himself is free, and in that sense is the alone (*kevala*).

In the *Yoga Sūtras* the term freedom (*moksha*) is not used for this great attainment, or great experience, or great discovery; the word aloneness (*kaivalya*) is used, which is seen to mean independence when applied to God, and therefore must mean the same when applied to the perfect yogi. The dictionaries give 'oneness' also as a meaning of this word, and its relation to the word for 'one' (*eka*) confirms this rendering. The meaning of unity will be discussed in a later chapter, but here we may note that at least it implies entire non-antagonism towards the world, and entire non-conflict within the yogi's own mind.

A God such as we have defined cannot be thought of as someone *having* freedom, since that someone would have to be something of the nature of the things and beings who are not free. In this case there can be no 'owner and owned': the two must be one. Such a yogi also is free, because he sees that all things which have troubled or have pleased him are there with his full approval, because he understands their value and use for the removal of the error he has been making all his life in allowing himself to come into bondage to them. They are part of his yogic path. He is not unlike the successful Stoic, who could say that nothing happened contrary to his will. He is also in line with an enlightened Christian who might say that not a sparrow falls to the ground without that 'father'. He sees that whatever is is best for the present moment. Yet he is the last man to leave it as it is.

We have considered circumstances. Among them we have to include the body itself. To the yogi the body is an 'instrument'. It is a tool for the contact of his mind with the world. In his novitiate it is highly probable that for him the pleasures of the mind already rank much higher than the pleasures of the body. Since people have not usually an equal activity of thinking, feeling, and willing, there have arisen schools of yoga teaching which provide for the special types of mind, in which one or other of these three may predominate. Typical schools are the Vedanta, with knowledge as its chief part, aim, and method, the *Bhagavad Gītā*, with its 'welfare of the world' doctrine of goodness and devotion, and the *Yoga Sūtras* of Patanjali, in which the will is used to govern both mind and body. All these three typical schools of yoga are intended to lead to the same goal, but by different paths. All start at the periphery of everyday experience, and end in the same experience of unity.

As the student proceeds he finds that the mind also becomes an instrument – 'the inner instrument' – and the pleasures of the mind become decreasingly important, while the spiritual aim comes more and more into view. Then, just as before there was the realization that body and circumstances cannot help one on the yogic way, so now there is the realization that the mind cannot help. Then, however, the formula has again to be remembered: 'Enough is necessary.' Death of the mind will not help, any more than death of the body. The aspirant must be alive. The spirit speaks to the mind, however, and says: 'Having your mind on me, you shall come to my state beyond.'[1] Is there a suggestion here that the mind 'does the trick'? The appearance of such a thing is quite misleading. The idea is that all things of the body and senses, and all states and activities of the mind are merely phenomena, temporary playthings, just as a little girl playing with a doll gets nothing from the doll but awakens her own capacity by what she does in the course of the playing.

1. *Bhagavad Gītā.*

CHAPTER 2

THE GOAL OF YOGA

A VERY large number of people in Western lands have heard or read of *nirvāna*. This has become in fact a regular word of the English language, defined in dictionaries variously as the cessation of desire and craving, the annihilation of personality, the transcendence of all states of body and mind, a state of complete understanding or bliss. As the Sanskrit verb *nir-vā* means 'to blow out' (as, e.g., a candle), the emphasis is sometimes put upon annihilation, when it is overlooked that the philosophy of life in which nirvana is a technical term is specifically aiming at the removal of ignorance and craving.

In old Indian literature the word nirvana occurs mostly in the Buddhist books. The following is an extract from Sir Edwin Arnold's *The Light of Asia*, which aims to present the life and teachings of Buddha as understood by a Southern Buddhist.

> If he who liveth, learning whence woe springs,
>   Endureth patiently, striving to pay
> His utmost debt for ancient evils done
>   In Love and Truth alway;
>
> If making none to lack, he throughly purge
>   The lie and lust of self forth from his blood;
> Suffering all meekly, rendering for offence
>   Nothing but grace and good;
>
> If he shall day by day dwell merciful,
>   Holy and just and kind and true; and rend
> Desire from where it clings with bleeding roots,
>   Till love of life have end:
>
> He – dying – leaveth as the sum of him
>   A life-count closed, whose ills are dead and quit,
> Whose good is quick and mighty, far and near,
>   So that fruits follow it.

No need hath such to live as ye name life;
  That which began in him when he began
Is finished: he hath wrought the purpose through
  Of what did make him Man.

Never shall yearnings torture him, nor sins
  Stain him, nor ache of earthly joys and woes
Invade his safe eternal peace; nor deaths
  And lives recur. He goes

Unto Nirvana. He is one with Life,
  Yet lives not. He is blest, ceasing to be.
Om, mani padme, hom! the Dewdrop slips
  Into the shining sea!

.   .   .   .   .

... Nay, there are those who surely pass
  Living and visible to utmost goal
By Fourth Stage of the Holy ones — the Buddhs
  And they of stainless soul.

Lo! Like fierce foes slain by some warrior,
  Ten sins along these Stages lie in dust,
The Love of Self, False Faith, and Doubt are three,
  Two more, Hatred and Lust.

Who of these Five is conqueror hath trod
  Three stages out of Four, yet there abide
The Love of Life on earth, Desire for Heaven,
  Self-Praise, Error and Pride.

As one who stands on yonder snowy horn
  Having nought o'er him but the boundless blue.
So, these sins being slain, the man is come
  Nirvana's verge unto.

Him the Gods envy from their lower seats;
  Him the Three Worlds in ruin should not shake;
All life is lived for him, all deaths are dead;
  Karma will no more make

New houses. Seeking nothing, he gains all;
  Foregoing self, the Universe grows 'I';
If any teach Nirvana is to cease,
  Say unto such they lie.

If any teach Nirvana is to live,
  Say unto such they err; not knowing this,
Nor what light shines beyond their broken lamps,
  Nor lifeless, timeless, bliss.

Enter the Path! There is no grief like Hate!
  No pains like passions, no deceit like sense!
Enter the Path! Far hath he gone whose foot
  Treads down one fond offence.

Enter the Path! There spring the healing streams
  Quenching all thirst! there bloom th' immortal flowers
Carpeting all the way with joy! there throng
  Swiftest and sweetest hours.

And at the conclusion of the whole poem comes the joyous chant of the Buddhist aspirant depicted as the author of the poem:

The Dew is on the lotus! – rise, Great Sun!
And lift my leaf and mix me with the wave.
Om mani padme hum, the Sunrise comes!
The Dewdrop slips into the shining Sea![1]

These verses represent the Hindu views of nirvana or liberation quite as well as the Buddhist views. They are quoted here because never elsewhere have the essentials been so fully or so happily expressed.

The nirvana thus presented may be regarded as very well expressing the goal of yoga. The word yoga means 'union' – as indicated in the expression 'the universe grows I'. This leaves no room for the assumption that 'The dewdrop slips into the shining sea' means complete annihilation.

After all, in our thought, in our present condition of environment and body and mind, 'annihilation' can mean nothing to us except the absence of our old familiar condition. What the new condition may be, if indeed it may rightly be called new or condition at all, being beyond time-process (and, incidentally, space-process, or extensity,

1. *op. cit.*, Bk VIII. *The Light of Asia* was written over seventy-five years ago.

as well) will be unknown to us until we achieve the 'illumination' which Buddha himself achieved, which led to his saying:

> I, Buddh, who wept with all my brothers' tears,
>   Whose heart was broken by a whole world's woe,
> Laugh and am glad, for there is Liberty.
>   Ho! ye who suffer! know
>
> Ye suffer from yourselves. None else compels,
>   None other holds you that ye live and die,
> And whirl upon the wheel, and hug and kiss
>   Its spokes of agony,
>   Its tire of tears, its nave of nothingness.[1]

In these words we find the former Gautama speaking of himself as Buddha, the enlightened.

Buddha, the title he now adopted, means 'enlightened'. It is understood that a Buddha is not a being who *has* enlightenment. We have to say that he *is* the light of enlightenment. Even with ourselves – men still on the way – we are not someone who has knowledge; we *are* the knowing, and indeed on close examination of ourselves, we find ourselves to be only 'knowing knowing knowing', as explained in my *Yoga Dictionary*.[2] This agrees, does it not, with the statement already quoted which declares it wrong to say that nirvana is to cease, or to live, and yet permits the expression 'lifeless, timeless bliss'?

All this is, of course, in accordance with the testimonies of many spiritual teachers and saints and sages in many lands who have spoken of the experience of unaccountable bliss and peace in the midst of ordinary scenes and affairs. It might be that lesser persons occasionally have an experience of an uplift which is nothing better than a nicer specimen of the same class of feelings that they had before – an answer, indeed, to their desire. Hence is the aspirant warned against *seeking* bliss. In the very seeking he has formulated to himself from his ignorance the nature of the bliss which can fulfil

---

1. *ibid.*, VIII.   2. Wood, Ernest, *Yoga Dictionary.*

his desire, and thereby has shut himself out from the supernal new experience. That new experience will nevertheless be the result of his endeavours to lead the good and pure life in thought as well as deed, with mastery of the mind as well as the body inasmuch as, though he cannot *produce* the illumination in the manner in which he can produce material articles and even states of mind, he has 'removed the clouds' which obscure the face of the true sun.

Still, it must not be thought that the word nirvana is confined to Buddhist scriptures, or Buddhist philosophy and religion. In that most famous of all Hindu scriptures, the *Bhagavad Gītā*, believed by the Hindus to be much older than the teaching of Buddha, the word nirvana occurs several times:

Verses 24–6 in Chapter or Discourse v read:

He whose happiness is within, whose delight is within, and likewise whose light even is within – that yogi, being of the nature of Brahman, goes up into the nirvana of Brahman.

For those strivers who are disassociated from desire and anger, whose intelligence is controlled, whose (real) selves are known, near is the nirvana of Brahman.

Verses 71–2 in Discourse II read:

The man who lives without longing, having cast off desires, without possessiveness, without egotism – he attains peace. This is the Brahmic state. Having obtained this, one is not confused. Being established in this at the end of (one's) time, one reaches even the nirvana of Brahman.

And verse 15, Discourse VI, reads:

The yogi, with mind controlled, always meditating thus on the Self (*ātmā*), arrives at my state, nirvanic ultimate, which is peace.

Here, however, we have a qualification of the word nirvana, in the term 'the Nirvana of Brahman'.

This calls for inspection of the ideas attached to Brahman in this Scripture.

That the *Bhagavad Gītā* is the great scripture of yoga in the eyes of the Hindu people is testified by the 'headings' which appear at the end of every Chapter or Discourse. It has eighteen chapters, and every one of them is described in these headings as dealing with a particular kind of yoga. Examples are the Yoga of Action, the Yoga of Devotion, the Yoga of Renunciation, the Yoga of Knowledge, the Yoga of the Divine Glories. In the text we meet frequently with such compounds as *sānkhya-yoga*, *buddhi-yoga*, and *ātma-yoga*.

In all these chapters the aim of yoga is described to much the same effect, though in various ways. At all stages it means allegiance to something high, and the yogi who adheres to a high principle is called '*yukta*' – united with or yoked to that principle. Thus one may be called *buddhi-yukta* if he has vowed to himself that he will adhere to the principle named *buddhi*, which is the wisdom of valuing for the advancing Self all the things and actions as they come along. In practice the successive yogas form a staircase, as it were, but when one comes to the top, having achieved a perfectly harmonious human condition, there is then not another step but a new platform of being, which is at the same time a release from the labours and limitations of the stairway. At the same time it is self-realization, or the discovery of one's own true nature.

This idea of liberation into a new sort of being or life has already been indicated in the references to the nirvana of Brahman. 'Coming to me' – the spirit speaking – 'entering my being', and 'reaching the beyond' are various expressions of the same idea. Here we have a statement of something beyond both body and mind, the understanding of which makes impossible both the kinds of anthropomorphism – of the body and of the mind – which are common among unphilosophic people, when they think of liberation, or heaven, or the Kingdom of God.

One read lately in the work of an eminent scientist, 'The world now looks to us more like a great mind than a great machine'. It is common, too, for people to attribute to 'God' (whom they have not seen) qualities and functions of mind such as thoughts, feelings, and purpose. But this should not be. 'Like a great mind' is another anthropomorphism.

Here are some of the quotations from the *Bhagavad Gītā* alluding to the Beyond:

He who thus truly knows my divine birth and action, having abandoned the body (at death), does not come to birth again. He comes to me. Many from whom passion, fear, and anger have gone, who are composed of me, who have resorted to me, who are purified by the knowledge-effort, have come into my being.

And what fruit of goodness is assigned to (the study of) the Vedas, to the sacrifices, to the austerities, and to the gifts – the yogi having known all this goes beyond it, and he attains the primal state beyond.

Be me-minded, devotee of me, sacrificer to me. Do reverence to me. To you shall come, with the self thus united, with me as (your) abode Beyond.

To those who are always united (and) serving I give along with love that *buddhi-yoga* by which they come to me.

Not by the scriptures, nor by austerity, nor by gift, nor by sacrificial offering can I be seen thus, as you have seen me. But by devotion, with no other object, I am able in such a manner truly to be known and to be seen, and to be entered into. My devotee, who has me as his supreme interest, who does actions for me, with attachment given up, without enmity in (the case of) all beings, he comes to me.

He whose (very) being is Brahman, himself serene, does not grieve (and) does not crave (anything). The same towards all beings, he obtains the supreme devotion to me. By (that) devotion he knows me truly; he enters that (state) without delay. Always doing all actions (while) also having his resort in me, by my grace he obtains the eternal unchanging goal (*padam*).

Go only to him for refuge, with all your being. Through his grace you will attain the peace Beyond, the eternal state.[1]

The definition of God in the *Yoga Sūtras* of Patanjali well indicates the same idea. In this case God is called *Īshwara*, which is, literally, the Ruler or Lord. After stating that attentiveness to God is one of the ways to the highest meditation and contemplation, Patanjali, the author, defines God as being unaffected by the afflictions which beset other

1. *Bhagavad Gītā*, iv, 9, 10; viii, 28; ix, 34; x, 10; xi, 53–5; xviii, 54–6, 62.

beings, the chief of which is ignorance, or by actions and their consequences.[1]

Putting alongside this the statement in the *Bhagavad Gītā* that the Supreme Being established the soul (*jivātmā*) with an eternal share of himself, and that such share becomes the lord *in each*, we see that the aspirant working towards independence (*kaivalya*) or freedom (*moksha*) is reaching to the same state of unaffectedness as is ascribed to the Lord (*Īshwara*). It is further stated that the yogi who makes the necessary efforts sees the *Īshwara* (the share aforementioned) in himself.[2]

After this it is easy to understand that the Beyond (*para*) is what is beyond both the things of the body and the functions of the mind, for these have not the characteristic of independence. Everything in the world is dependent upon other things in many ways – the body needing air and food, to mention only two necessities. The mind is equally dependent, for where would hearing, touch, sight, taste, and smell be without objects, where would thought or inference be without objects, and where would even love be without a beloved?

Perhaps the best way to understand the Beyond is to picture body and mind as equal partners, side by side:

ether				
air				will
fire	}	Body	Mind {	feeling
water				thought
earth				

These two are reacting on each other all the time. Even when the mind immersed in an act of mental reflection is not attentive to the body, it nevertheless works with pictures taken from outside into the memory and with thoughts based upon them.

The *two together* constitute the 'flow of dependent origination'[3] or causal law so emphatically alluded to by Buddha.

1. *Yoga Sūtras*, i, 23–4; ii, 3.   2. *Bhagavad Gītā*, xv, 7–11.
3. *Pratītyasamutpāda*.

Causality is certainly not of the material alone. On this point it is most important to observe that there are in the world three potencies:

> variety
> harmony
> unity

In studying the principle of variety, we find that all the substances of Nature defend their individuality to some extent. In the main the chemical substances are very individualistic. As declared in what is called the Vaisheshika philosophy of old India, each one shows not only substance, but also qualities and actions. A piece of iron, e.g., will bubble when it contacts certain acids, but a piece of gold will not do so. In such ways all things show *personality*, even as a human being does in a more complicated way. That 'personality' is the basis of variety, or perhaps we should say is the principle upholding variety in the world.

Then the mind comes in, and in all its constructive affairs operates the principle of harmony, as when a man guides his legs with his eyes and guides his eyes with his legs. In this way eyes are for walking and legs for seeing, and indeed every function of the body serves every other, with the solitary exception of the sex organs and other reproductive apparatus, which operate for the sake of another being or body. And when the mind plans a clock or a motor-car it operates harmony, because it takes things which are separate and puts them together in such a manner that there is mutual help instead of mere separateness or even conflict. In what we commonly call feeling (seen primitively in interestedness, and more advancedly in ethical love) we have again harmony-making.

The intelligent mind more and more serves harmony, and indirectly even the unity which harmony serves, and indeed the instinct of self-preservation found in the most primitive organisms is an expression of this principle or power of unity.

Well, then, from these considerations we can see that

both matter and mind, having 'dependent origination' as the Buddhists describe it, are not of the nature of the Beyond. The Beyond is, in fact, frequently alluded to as 'That' in Hindu scriptures, in contradistinction to 'This', which contains both body and mind.

The word for Beyond (*para*) could also be translated as 'other than'. In both cases we have to beware of the ascription of any relativity between 'That' and 'This'. The Beyond has no relation whatever to 'This', for the simple reason that the beyondness of it takes it outside the sphere of any relativity or comparison whatsoever.

It is for this reason that the ascription of 'emptiness' or 'voidness' (terms used in some schools of thought) are quite invalid if applied to the Beyond, as the ultimate pair of opposites – presence and absence, fullness and emptiness, facts and space – are both transcended.

The 'That' or the Beyond therefore cannot be 'higher' than the two, also cannot be 'above', and thus *not being in a series* cannot again be transcended with a *regressus infinitus*.

The word 'reality' is probably the best term to name that Beyond, for if we ask ourselves what it is that both being and non-being, or both presence and absence, have in common, we can only say 'reality'. Reality is a good word for this, as it is the same as 'royalty'. Royalty is properly conceived as above the law – something beyond the categories of being and non-being, in this case.

God, also, is quite a good word, *if we remember* that it means this reality or fundamental Independence. The word can then be for us a word of discovery, not a word of definition. In science we have words of definition, but here we have a word with which to give *direction* to the mind, a word which is like a boat, such as Columbus used when he set out to discover something that he did not know.

Now that we have defined the goal of yoga as the discovery of the indefinable, we have to ask two more questions:

How can man, with either mind or body, make that discovery?

Are there lesser goals also for which men practise yoga?

The answer to the second question is 'yes', and we shall come to a study of those in due course in this book.

The answer to the first is that he *can* make the discovery because he already has in himself that which is beyond both mind and body, even when he has not yet learned to be attentive to it. On this account the goal of yoga is often spoken of as 'self-realization', the meaning being that neither the body nor the mind is the self.

The standard and most authoritative work on Yoga, the *Yoga Sūtras* of Patanjali, alludes to the goal of yoga as *kaivalya*, which may be translated as either 'the state of oneness' or 'independence'. The latter term seems good because the same book defines *Īshwara* or God, as we have already remarked, as a specific sort of spirit (*purusha*) who is free in the sense of not depending on anything else, i.e. God has independent origination and existence.

The aphorisms (*sūtras*) expressing this independence are as follows:

Or, it (i.e. the non-cognitive Contemplation) comes from Attentiveness to God.

God is a particular soul, unaffected by containers of sources of trouble (i.e. bodies), works and (their) fruition.[1]

The yogi meditating on this idea acquires the same state, which is then described as *kaivalya*, which is brought about by his consequent disjunction of his sense of I from all the things of the body and the functions of the mind upon which he was theretofore dependent. The dependence was, however, of his own creation, inasmuch as he had been allowing himself to be psychologized or fascinated by them. The statements about Independence are:

When the seeds of bondage have been destroyed by his (the

1. *Yoga Sūtras*, i, 23–4. 'God is the perfect spirit' would probably be a better translation, and quite literal for the Sanskrit *purusha vishesha*, since *purusha* is the spirit beyond all manifestation (*prakriti*), including both matter and mind, and *vishesha* means most excellent as well as specific. In translating the term as 'particular soul' in my book, *Practical Yoga: Ancient and Modern*, I was too much influenced by earlier translators.

yogi's) being uncoloured even by the pure mind, there will be Independence.

Independence is the counter-product when the qualities of nature are devoid of purpose for the real man, or (when) the power of consciousness stands firm in its own nature.[1]

It is necessary to say a few words here about the nature of time. Time is seen where the mind or its products are at work. If nothing ever changed, would there be time? Some would answer 'Yes, although each moment would be exactly like the previous one'. But really that would only be a state of complete materiality. Matter – fundamental matter or materiality – is inertia, that which does not change. That is what the chemists were looking for, and for a while thought they had, in the shape of the chemical atoms.

The physicists have learnt from their experience – once bitten, twice shy – and do not dare to assume fundamentality even for their electrons, which anyhow are more like force (change) than matter. Even latent or potential force – well conceived in these days – is matter in the sense of 'something here', although an infinite amount of it, or a head of power, may theoretically be present in a point of space. But wherever mind is there is either change or the potential of change, the power of change. Material objects may continue without change, but thought is an operation which implies change and sequence. If it is said that even the minerals and the chemical elements are very slowly, imperceptibly slowly, changing on their own initiative, we shall have to credit them with a very primitive degree of personality and subscribe to the idea that wherever matter is mind also is.

Independence is a great mystery, as being fundamental and different from all combinations and interactions, for there is not dependency without independence. There must be a core of independence for anything to be acted upon. This is well seen, as the present writer has pointed out in several of

1. Quoted from Wood, Ernest, *Practical Yoga: Ancient and Modern.* Aphorisms i, 34; i, 49.

his books, particularly *The Glorious Presence*, when we consider a system or group of mutually dependent articles – a group of planets, for example. In such a group, named, let us say, A to Z, any one of them is dependent upon the other twenty-five. They are all pulling it and pushing it all the time so that in the final balance of A, whether in the pose of rest or that of motion, it is what it is and does what it does under the power of those other twenty-five.

But here comes the important point and the hub of the mystery: that one named A is one of the twenty-five pushers and pullers in relation to any other one (B to Z). Therefore *everything and everyone has a share of the original power*, in all relational respects.

Can we become conscious of that power, and be aware of it, not merely of the pushings and pullings to which we are responding constantly? The yogi says we can, or at least he can, and when he discovers it he has found peace. Power is always peace – it is the machinery that makes the fuss.

This knowing of independence is an illumination and a mystery. What does the water-lily plant know of the sunshine and air, and of its own flowering in that ambience? Yet, while still in the root in the mud and while still in the stem in the water it displays the impulse by which it takes itself to that goal. It is true – what the poets feel – that in standing and in walking and even in lying down we in some degree float, to the extent of our share of the original power. The apple that falls to the ground also lifts the earth. This is true of the mind as well as the body. Without that independence there would be no response, no knowing, for at base there is no such thing as the completely passive reception of modifications in consciousness.

This independence *is the Self*. To know this as the Self is the goal of the yogi. This Self cannot but be of the same nature as the original power. In the *Bhagavad Gītā* it is precisely expressed as such:

A share of myself, having become an eternal living being in the world of living beings, attracts the sense-organs, of which mind is the sixth, which are situated in Nature.

(This) master (*Īshwara*), who (thus) obtains a body and who also goes beyond it (at death), having grasped these (senses) goes his way, just as the wind (takes) scents from their resting-places.

Having governed the ear, the eye, the organs of touch and taste, and smell, and the mind, he makes use of the objects of sense.

The deluded do not perceive him (thus) joined with the qualities of Nature (*gunas*), whether he is departing or staying still, or enjoying (the senses). They see, whose eye is knowledge.

Yogis, striving, also see him, instated in themselves. The inattentive who have not disciplined themselves, even though striving, do not see him.[1]

Or, as Emerson put it:

> Substances at base divided
> In their summits are united;
> There the holy essence rolls,
> One through separated souls.

and

> Ever fresh the broad creation,
> A divine improvisation,
> From the heart of God proceeds,
> A single will, a million deeds.

It is in this aim of Independence that the goal of yoga is at one with the Freedom (*moksha*) which is the goal of the Vedanta philosophy, the nirvana of Buddha, and the Kingdom of the teachings of Jesus. Another form of yoga practice (though not called such by its votaries) is *Zen*, a word derived from the Sanskrit *dhyāna* through the Chinese *chan*. This school (or rather group of schools, for there are minor differences) was prepared for in China by the Indian Buddhist monk Bodhidharma early in the sixth century. For nine years he practised meditation 'like a wall', which we may take to mean not responding to external impressions during meditation, at the Shorinji Temple in North China, and in course of time his method was carried to Japan and established there under the name *Zen*.

1. *Bhagavad Gītā* xv, 7–11. Trans. by Ernest Wood in *The Bhagavad Gītā Explained*. There are many translations – probably a hundred – of the *Gītā* into the English language.

This is definitely, by definition, a school of Buddhist meditation, though it derives not from any verbal teachings or instructions given by Buddha, but from 'a special transmission (by Buddha) outside the Scriptures, with no dependence on words and letters'. It is related that on a certain occasion a flower was presented to Buddha with a request to state the *Dharma*. Buddha simply held up the golden flower and gazed at it in silence. One of the disciples, the Venerable Mahakasyapa, caught the idea (no, we must not call it that!) which could not be spoken, nor even thought, and was transported with joy. That radiance then became transmissible from one to another, as one candle lights another – in this case if the other is ready for it. But the radiance is everywhere, and so the method of *Zen* postulates an endeavour and promises an achievement attainable by the 'meditation' with no mind, which is no-mind. This is achieved, according to some of its teachers, by means of mind-baffling statements (*koans*) to be tackled by the aspirants in meditation, or by startling non-logical assertive questions (*mondos*) to which the disciple must instantaneously respond. These are problems which life sets us all the time, so the disciple must at all times and in all circumstances face everything with this beyond-the-mind faculty, if we may be pardoned for so or in any way describing or alluding to it. It is indescribable, and there is no distinction between knower and known (no such duality). Even subject-self is overcome. The resulting experience or condition is called *satori*. It conforms to Buddha's teaching that the last of the 'fetters' to go is Ignorance or Error, the conceiving of oneself as anything conceivable.

It is thus seen that the 'goal' is the same for all, whether Yogis, Vedantins, Christians, Zenists. To this list we should add the Sufis, with their stages of awakening, purification, illumination, and union or identification, which is achieved by completely self-forgetting devotional love, so that it could be said that when the union is gained the man is not lost and yet only God goes on.

Still, as we have already said, the majority of aspirants are inclined to postpone this ultimate goal for later times (although they know that the light of it illumines all the way) and content themselves with lesser goals. The lesser goals of the practices of yoga may be easily listed:

Peace of mind and heart.
Power of the will, and of love and intellect.
Direct influence of the mind upon the body and the world outside the body.
Psychic faculties of various kinds.
Control of mind and power of concentration.
Control of the emotions – removal of worry, pride, anger, fear, lust, and greed.
Bodily health, suppleness, beauty, and longevity.
The complete prevention and removal of psychosomatic dangers and troubles.

CHAPTER 3

THE ETHICS AND MORALITY OF YOGA

IT will probably come as a surprise to many to learn that
progress in yoga depends upon goodness in personal character and in social relations, and that this is, indeed, laid down
authoritatively as the first requisite in the main-line system
of yoga, namely, the *Yoga Sūtras* of Patanjali.

In the *Yoga Sūtras* eight limbs (*angas*) or tools or aids are
prescribed. These are sometimes spoken of as 'steps', because
the course of yoga practice is often alluded to as a road
(*mārga*) or path or way.

The following is a list of the eight 'limbs', in order,
though it is intended in the present chapter to draw particular attention to only the first two. The others are listed
merely to give a preview of the other six, to which they lead.
The eight are:

1. Abstention (*Yama*).
2. Observance (*Niyama*).
3. Posture (*Āsana*).
4. Breath-control (*Prānāyāma*).
5. Sense-withdrawal (*Pratyāhāra*).
6. Concentration (*Dhāranā*).
7. Meditation (*Dhyāna*).
8. Contemplation (*Samādhi*).[1]

It will be noticed that the first two of these eight are concerned with the aspirant's attitude towards the outer world
and towards himself, in short, to ethics and morality in the
widest sense of those terms; the next three have to do with
the body and the senses; and the last three deal with the
mind. Really, the transactions of life are between the real
man (*purusha*) or Self (*ātmā*) and the world, but there are two
instruments in between, as it were – the mind as inner

1. *Yoga Sūtras*, ii, 29.

instrument and the body as outer instrument. These two tools – or perhaps we should call them kits, as they are both quite complex – have to be put into good order and kept in good order as part of the regular system of conditioning.

Now to the Abstentions and Observances:

Abstention, says the text of the *Yoga Sūtras*, consists of five self-restraints, described as (1) non-injury, (2) truthfulness, (3) non-theft, (4) spiritual conduct, and (5) non-greed. The ideal is to maintain these five in all circumstances and at all times.

The would-be student may be somewhat staggered by this demand at the outset, but if he confesses this to his teacher (*guru*) the following conversation is likely to ensue:

Teacher. Yes, I admit these are difficult to carry out perfectly. But tell me, can you say that you have entirely given up the *desire* to injure, to lie, to steal, to be sensual, and to be greedy? Is it a pleasure to you to think of injuring, lying, dishonesty, sensuality, and greed?

Pupil. Yes, I can truly say that I do not *want* these impulses. I do not do these things for pleasure, but through either force of habit or temptation I do them occasionally.

Teacher. Well, if you have given up the *desire* to injure anybody or to lie or steal or be sensual or greedy, and have given up pleasure in the *thought* of injury to another, etc., the battle is already almost won. You may proceed.

The second step, Observance, is also described as five-fold, but this time the five are things to do, whereas the first step listed things not to do.

They are: 1. Cleanliness (*Shaucha*).
   2. Contentment (*Santosha*).
   3. Austerity (*Tapas*).
   4. Self-study (*Swādhyāya*).
   5. Attentiveness to God (*Ïshwara-pranidhāna*).[1]

Cleanliness is usually described as having reference to both mind and body – in thought, word, and deed. The word for contentment (*santosha*) comes from a verbal root, *tush*,

1. *Yoga Sūtras*, ii, 32.

which means to be pleased, so this virtue is something more than mere passive contentedness. It does not imply passivity or resignation, but is allied to the doctrine of equanimity (*samatwa*) much emphasized in the *Bhagavad Gītā*. Speaking of the advanced yogi, it says:

He excels who has sameness of appreciation (or valuation – *buddhi*) towards well-wishers, friends, enemies, strangers, neutrals, haters, and kinsmen, and even saints and sinners.[1]

Another verse speaks of him as regarding a lump of earth, a rock, or gold as the same. It states that he is also perfectly poised amidst cold and heat, pleasure and pain, respect and contumely. And why so? Because he is satisfied with knowledge and experience, and above all with the Self within. Because he recognizes the value of all these things for the inner man he is not only not emotionally upset, but he is positively pleased. It does not mean that he is physically insensitive to cold and heat (though yoga practices in connexion with breathing and relaxation do make him very adaptable in this respect) but that his emotional attitude is calm.

As the path of yoga is one of definite endeavours, as listed in the remaining six limbs (*angas*), it should be clearly understood that the aspirant is accepting gladly all the adverse circumstances that arise, regarding them as opportunity, instead of lamenting the situation. It is similar to the doctrine of the Stoic, Epictetus, who declared, 'There is only one thing for which God has sent me into the world, and that is to develop every kind of virtue or strength, and there is nothing in all the world that I cannot use for this purpose.'

Further, it is generally believed that the circumstances which arrive 'without effort' – which means not as the result of our immediate or recent action – are not purely accidental, but are related to our defects and merits of character, on account of which we did some actions in the past – even in past lives – which have caused this experience now. This is quite akin to a modern view expressed by the first Henry

1. *Bhagavad Gītā*, vi, 9.

Ford. When being interviewed by a news reporter he happened to remark that he never made a mistake. The reporter, surprised, asked for an explanation, and was told, 'Of course, I have done many things ignorantly and sometimes without sufficient thought, but I learned from those actions, and would not have learned otherwise, so they were not fundamentally mistakes.'

In India there is also a definite doctrine of 'fate' with regard to events which is expounded in the *Bhagavad Gītā*. There the teacher says:

Learn from me the five lines of causation (which appear) in the achievement of every action, as stated in the concluding portion of the *sānkhya* (philosophy): (1) The site for it; (2) the doer of it; (3) the different kinds of instruments used in it; (4) the various different kinds of functions (or motions) employed; and (5) the divinity (or fate). Whatever action a man undertakes – whether in the right way or in the wrong way – these five are the causes of it.[1]

It may not occur to the reader at first glance, but the fifth of these reasons always comes in. The average Hindu is therefore in accord with the statement of Robert Burns, that 'the best laid schemes o' mice and men gang aft agley'. More than that, we may always expect an unseen (*adrishta*) element to come in, which may in fact upset a good plan or, on the other hand, bring a bad one to a successful conclusion.

Such unseen and incalculable elements are 'those which arrive without effort' (*prāptas*). The Western person is often annoyed when something 'accidental' spoils his work or his plans. The Oriental expects it, or at least is not surprised by it, and so accepts it without anger or resentment. He attributes it to the unseen, which, being beyond mind – beyond the most perfect planning – is of the *deva* nature, or the gods, but still within the field of causation, the result of some karma, or action previously done.

Whether it is an adverse 'accident' (i.e. unseen factor) or a propitious one, still the yogi is pleased (*santushta*) with

1. *ibid.*, xviii, 13–15.

it. The mistake will henceforth be corrected; the man, having gone through the experience with contentment and attentiveness, has learned his lesson and had his awakening – a lesson he would not have had without the experience, and which he could only have anticipated and averted with much thought and wisdom.

Next – the third of the five Observances – comes austerity (*tapas*). This does not mean self-mortification – a mistake made by many. How could self-mortification lead on to good posture, good breathing, control of the senses, concentration, meditation, and contemplation? On the contrary, the *Bhagavad Gītā* says:

Yoga is not for the excessive eater, nor for one who avoids food too intently; not for one addicted to excessive sleep, nor to (excessive) wakefulness. Yoga becomes the destroyer of pain for one whose food and recreations are yogic, whose efforts in actions are yogic, whose sleeping and waking are yogic.[1]

Much light is thrown by the succeeding verses upon the use of the term 'yogic'. It could also be translated 'proper to the occasion' to convey the meaning, for it is when the lower mind mechanism is directed to thoughts about the Self, without longings for objects of desire, that it can be called yogic. In such a case there will not be excess or any unnaturalness or unhealthy habits. The Self has now become the main interest, or in more modern terms it is the welfare of the inner man on his path of evolution or unfoldment that is the subject of thought and interest.

The culmination of this group of verses comes when the yogi is described as so much united with the Self that he 'absorbs the unlimited happiness of contact with Brahman'. Then, when he realizes that there is the same Self (*ātmā*) 'standing in all beings everywhere, and all beings existing in that Self' – the same everywhere, regardless of pleasure and pain – that yogi is considered to be the highest.

In the same work there is as much condemnation of self-mortification as of over-indulgence:

1. *ibid.*, vi, 16.

Those people who inflict upon themselves fierce austerity (*ghora tapas*) ... unintelligent ... suppressing the groups of (small) beings in their bodies, and me (the spirit) also established within the body – know them as having demoniac resolves.[1]

This is confirmed by a description of the foods that are good and are liked by the people whose taste is pure, as 'those which increase vitality, bodily harmony, strength, health, pleasure, and gratification, and are juicy, oily, firm, and heartening'[2].

The *Yoga Sūtras* are also very clear on this point – that austerity (*tapas*) does not mean injury to the body.

From *tapas*, with the decline of impurity, come the powers (or perfections; *siddhis*) of the body and the organs (of sense and action), and: 'Excellence of the body consists of correct form, beauty, strength, and very firm well-knitness'.[3]

The last word (*vajra-sanhananatwa*) though usually regarded as referring to hardness, could also mean 'great energy', for *vajra* means 'thunderbolt' as well as 'diamond', and *sanhananatwa* means 'mightiness' or 'powerfulness'.

Enough has been said to show that austerity (*tapas*) does not mean mortification, and must mean body-conditioning, with great firmness of will, avoiding all bodily indulgence and insisting upon that quantity and kind of food, exercise, and rest which one believes to be best for the body. This is, of course, good common sense also, leading to greater bodily health, pleasure, and happiness than can be obtained by thoughtlessness or weak indulgence.

To show that this attitude is not merely that of the *rāja-yoga* school, and of philosophic schools such as the *Bhagavad Gītā* represents, we will quote also from that most authoritative of *hatha-yoga* works, the *Hathayoga Pradīpikā*: 'Over-eating; effortful exertion; idle chatter; hard vows; needing to be with people; restlessness – by these six yoga is ruined.'[4]

Finally, that there may be no doubt whatsoever in this important matter, we will quote that most abstract of all philosophers, Shankarāchārya, he who over two thousand

1. *ibid.*, xvii, 5, 6.   2. *ibid.*, xvii, 8.   3. *Yoga Sūtras*, ii, 43; iii, 45.
4. *Hathayoga Pradīpikā*, i, 15.

years ago – according to orthodox belief – made India ring
with the One Reality (*adwaita*) doctrine:

Seat or posture is only that in which contemplation of Brahman
can be comfortable and continuous; that should be adopted, not
others which interfere with comfort.

Straightness of limbs occurs when there is resting in harmony with
Brahman, not if there is only straightness like a dried-up tree.

 Having achieved knowledge-sight, one sees the world as composed of Brahman – that kind of seeing is the highest, not the
gazing in front of the nose. Or when there is the cessation of (the
distinction of) seer, seeing, and seen, there is the *Steadiness of Vision*.[1]

Coming now to the fourth of the five Observances, Self-
study (*swādhyāya*), we will briefly say that it means there
should be some daily study bearing upon the nature of oneself – not merely study of outward or objective things. There
is plenty of difference of opinion about what study this
implies. Many maintain that it must refer to the study of
one's own scriptures, one's own religion; but the general
attitude of the *Sānkhya* philosophy which pervades the *Yoga
Sūtras* should discount this view. It is true that *swa* does
not mean 'self', but as a prefix means 'one's own' (e.g. *swa-
karma* means an action done by oneself; *swakula* means one's
own family; *swadesha* means one's own country). We shall
probably rightly take the meaning to be the study of what
really concerns oneself – on the principle that 'the proper
study of mankind is man', the study of one's own being and
nature, as distinguished from the study of external things,
which is usually pursued for some gain to the bodily life.

Finally, we come to the fifth of the Observances, attentiveness to God (*Īshwara pranidhāna*).

It is really problematical how one should regard the idea
of God as ruler (*Īshwara*) in the *Yoga Sūtras*. Usually the
first tendency is to think that one should feel devotion to the
Founder or the Basis of all known being – both matter and

1. *Aparokshānubhūti* (Direct Experience), by Shankarāchārya, verses
115 and 116, translated in Wood, Ernest, *The Glorious Presence*.

life. But to be grateful to God as Ruler is one thing, and to regard God as the model or archetype of one's own future state of being is another. The latter is the formulation in the meditative portion of the *Yoga Sūtras* – a matter already dealt with in our Chapter 2. The yogi must become unaffected by troubles – of which ignorance is the chief and the source of all – or by works and their effects outside or inside.[1]

In the meantime, however, he is to remember that this *Īshwara* is not an independent being withdrawn into himself by the possession of complete free will. It is the Master or Ruler of all who or which have not attained the same, and the ruler for their good, that is, the supreme Teacher. The implication of this combination of a supreme ruler and teacher is that no one can escape the benevolent lessons of life even for a moment, and therefore devotion is perfectly in order. The hand of God is in every event, and the constancy of it gives it the aspect of Law, even the 'laws of Nature'.

To receive all experience in the devotional spirit, knowing that the fruitage of the lesson comes after the experience, not before it, nor even during it, includes at once great faith and great love of God. We might conceivably – might we not? – have found ourselves in a perfectly hellish state of life in which there was only endless torment, disorder, and chance. How grand it is to be under this Rule, such that even the mind cannot fundamentally stray, and cannot miss the benefit even of its own errors. What grandness, what joy, to be under this rule, and even more to feel and understand that some day we shall be part of the ruling, not of the ruled, when our life will not be only permeated by the joy of the understanding of the Law as now, but will itself be the glory of the being of it.

Thus comes in 'Attentiveness to God', which is the acceptance of all experience without resentment or antagonism, not merely seeing the good in everything, but seeing the God in everything, which puts our emotions as

1. *Yoga Sūtras*, i, 23, 24, already quoted.

well as our understanding right. Such is the 'love of God' when that teachership is known.

The *Sūtras*, continuing their definition of God, further explain:

In That is the ultimate source of all knowledge.

That same was the Teacher of the ancients, not being limited by time.

Of That the expressor is the sacred syllable (*Om*).

There should be repetition of this, with pondering upon its meaning.[1]

These ethical and moral heights which are thus taught as the very beginning of the yoga path are announced not merely as leading to inward benefit. Their effects are stated to permeate the external living also. The benefits (which as they arise again contain new lessons) which the good receive – and what nonsense is this modern pose of being ashamed of goodness! – are announced in definite order, according to the list of ten, the two fives. These are briefly stated, so it is necessary for the student to interpret them, amplify them, and apply them to his own life by his own thought, and then, in due course, realize their magic.

When non-injury is accomplished, there will be abandonment of animosity in his presence.

When non-lying is accomplished, the results of actions become subservient to him.

When non-theft is accomplished, all jewels approach him.

When non-sensuality is accomplished, vigour is obtained.

When non-greed is accomplished, there arises perception of the method of births.

From (external) cleanliness arises protectiveness of the body and detachment from others.

And then, when there is mind-cleanliness, come (in order) high-mindedness, attentiveness (or one-pointedness), mastery of the senses, and fitness for the vision of the self.

From Contentment comes the obtaining of the highest form of pleasure.

From Body-conditioning, with the decline of impurity, come the powers of the body and the senses.

1. *ibid.*, i, 25–8.

From Self-study arises contact with the desired divinity.
From Attentiveness to God comes the power of contemplation.[1]

To appreciate these results of the ten virtues, or abstentions (*yamas*) and observances (*niyamas*), we need to understand the outlook and background of the Hindu mind of old
times, prior to the influx of modern machinery, mass production and mass education for material ends.

1. Non-injury. By the 'law of karma' no injury can come
in future to the non-injurer, except what comes as a result
of his injurious doings prior to his seeing and following the
true path. On this theory and belief people are receiving
what they have given or done to others. The blessing of this
law is also to be taken into account, for the lesson is at all
times appropriate to the person. If a person, for example,
robbed others in the past, perhaps with violence, it must
have been because he was insensitive to their suffering, and
now the repercussion of that upon himself may be expected
to make him feel what suffering is, with the result that in the
course of time he will feel it even when applying it to others.

This belief might fill people with the fear that they may
have an immense back-log of painful experience 'in the
bank' as it were, ready to pounce on them as an incalculable
or unseen factor in their present and future plans. But these
fears must be discounted for two reasons. One reason is the
fact that our lives are a mixture of pleasure and pain, of
what we may call good and bad, most of the time, which
shows that the incurring and the paying of these debts has
been and is being more or less equal all the time, so that
one cannot suppose oneself to have been a terrible monster
with a dreadful quantity and quality of sins behind one
(flattering to one's vanity as the thought may be). The other
reason against fear is the doctrine and belief that what we
now do with genuine unselfishness cancels out an equal
amount of old 'bad karma' which has not yet come into
effect in our present lives. The logic of this is that one has
somehow learnt the lesson by study and thought and wis-

---

1. *ibid.*, ii, 35-45.

dom, and does not need to learn it the hard way, but all the same pays off the old karma by the good actions one spontaneously does.

The aphorism on this subject goes a little further. The abandonment of animosity against oneself must of course come to an end with the exhaustion of the old collection of debts, but more comes in. There is the tendency for others to reform their ways in one's presence. It is good for us to see the good and to have the company of the good. Indeed, to be good is itself a good deed. In social relations this is a large part of the mutual benefit. Even the illustrations in the newspapers of the slender ladies who look so nice and surely are enjoying health and suppleness (although put there merely to persuade others to buy various articles) are part of our 'company of the good', which is so definitely thought of in India that it enjoys a special name – the *Satsanga*. This benefit is not from imitation, but from emulation, and it is both external and internal. Besides, how could anyone reach a high point of spiritual contemplation if his mind contained low and selfish thoughts?

2. The results of truthfulness are considered in the commentaries on the *Sūtras* to be due to truthfulness in both word and thought. The results of actions being subservient to us, translated into our own idiom, can only mean that henceforth we shall get what we work for. Why do people so often fail? Chiefly because they have been willing to live in a state of self-deception. They aim at health, for example, and do something about it, but still spoil the work by various prejudices against the good counsels which are available in the health and physical culture magazines. They will not give up . . . although they know it is harmful; they hope it will be all right, and surely just a little will not matter!

Again, people do not measure their karma (circumstances) against their strength. Good sense (truthfulness) would tell them that to be realistic and accept *what is*, without useless wishing and complaining, and then act according to their best judgement for a reasonable aim in the circumstances, measuring their own ability and strength realistically also, will mostly result in the desired success. But do they follow this good sense, this truthfulness to themselves in thought, first of all? No, they complain and fret, and poison the air for others as well as themselves.

Truthfulness in speech is the cement of friendship and social confidence, and whoever breaks that causes wide suspicion, as King Henry V explained with wonderful eloquence and effect in Shakespeare's play.

3. Jewels approach. It was natural for the simple-living people of India in the old days to think of jewels as wealth. There were no banks to give them interest on their deposited savings, and there was generally no thought of accumulating currency, which may perhaps have been in process of depreciation, then as now. Even today the Hindus generally regard the family jewels as their bank. But consider the law of karma as applied to riches. It could be formulated as 'what you earn you have' – for all time. But if you rob, you lose. If a child comes to birth 'with a silver spoon in his mouth' it is because he has earned it in the past. Origen, one of the Christian Church Fathers, had the same idea.

Many rich people dislike the idea of reincarnation, feeling how terrible it would be not to have their riches, and yet they must leave them behind when they die! Not a bit of it. If they have earned or deserved them they will be theirs in the future, always provided that they have not stolen them in any way, for in that case the jewels will not approach in the balancing of karma. So there *is*, after all, material as well as spiritual gain in holding to the virtues. There is, however, in the doctrine the clear notion that not all past karmas can be brought together at one time, or even in one lifetime or, more properly, bodytime. There is therefore an effect of the grouping into a type of lifetime of a certain number of compatible karmas. This being the case – that not all the karmas can be represented at one time, but only a compatible group – it could be possible for a well-to-do person to find himself in poverty for a while, even perhaps for a lifetime. Thus, as it was once put, 'The dead king may next see the light in a coolie's tent'.

A case which came within my own experience is to the point. A certain elderly blind man whom I knew well had for many years practised yoga under the direction of a *guru* known to both of us. This blind man told me that as a result of his yoga meditations he had become able to see into his previous life, which, he said, took place about seven hundred years ago. In that life, his story proceeded, he had been a small *rāja* (king) in northern India. While being kind to his family and those who pleased him, he had been harsh and sometimes dreadfully cruel to the poor cultivators and his enemies. The result of some of his acts of oppression and cruelty, he said, was his present blindness and poverty, which had, however, been a blessing in disguise, because they had caused him to become great friends with the poor villagers living round about, and so he had 'learnt real friendship in this life'. When the bad karma was paid off – he believed – he would be back again in a position of comparative wealth and influence, with the advantage of an improved character and disposition. I had, of course, no means of verifying the accuracy of his vision or memory of the past, but I did find that in ordinary matters he had remarkable clairvoyance and telepathic powers.

4. The word here translated 'non-sensuality' is *Brahmacharya*. *Charya* means 'conduct' or 'way of life'. Brahma here means roughly 'spiritual' or 'of the character of Brahman'. It is generally taken to mean celibate, though there are many who interpret it to mean that cohabitation may be indulged in, not however for bodily or emotional pleasure, but only as and when enjoined by the scriptures or when regarding the function as a sacred trust of power to ensure the future of humanity or of the family.

This 'way of life' is stated to lead to vigour. The belief among yogis is that abstention from the use of the sex function (which is often maintained after the duty to one's family has been successfully done) leads to a sublimation of the bodily energy, which would otherwise have been expended wastefully, into the functions and powers of the higher mind. It is argued – contrary to popular opinion in the West – that the sex function is the one function of the body which does not in any way contribute to the welfare of the body, but exists only for the benefit of others, that is, future generations. If abstention leads to any bodily disorder, that must be put down to the effect of wrong emotional attitudes towards the subject, and consequent wrong ideas. No doubt modern popular literature has created a vast amount of ignorant thinking and unhealthy opinion on the subject, and the human power of imagination has intensified the cravings of young people in the modern world far beyond the limits of naturalness.

This question will come up again in our chapter on the vital force of Kundalinī, where the yoga teaching is all in favour of abstention (when socially justified), and the direction of the vital forces to the 'higher' functions of life is quite elaborately described.

5. The word here translated 'non-greed' is *aparigraha*. It could also be translated 'non-covetousness', or literally, non-grasping (*graha*) all round or round about (*pari*). It is related to one of the five great troubles (*kleshas*) of human life – possessiveness (*abhinivesha*). The difference of meaning is that while *aparigraha* is concerned with grasping or getting, *abhinivesha* is more concerned with holding on to what one has. As to the latter, there is an aphorism which states that this trouble is so firmly grounded in human life that it is instinctive even with the wise.[1] The commentators have often emphasized that the chief part of it lies in clinging to the body – something usually very much overdone, the point of view of the yogis being that the body exists as a ground of living for the sake of spiritual attainments. Their position could also be summed up in the saying, 'It is better to lose your body and save your "soul" than to save your body and lose your "soul" ' – losing your soul meaning lowering your standard of life (which has nothing to do with 'standard of living', of course).

1. *ibid.*, ii, 9.

When this virtue is attained, says the aphorism, the yogi will have a perception of the method of births. In the first place he will see that it is not what we have but the use that we make of it that matters in life. So, as regards material things, the yogi is not much concerned with more acquisitions, or with the satisfaction of common desires. He becomes habituated mentally and emotionally to the idea of 'living on the wing' rather than 'digging in'. Many are the practising yogis who outside business hours and social duties are engaged in yoga. They are almost recognizable by the equanimity with which they meet and deal with 'what comes'. Later on, the advanced yogi renounces the plan-making faculty (*vikalpa*). He makes no plans for himself, but meets the karma that comes and attends to the calls of duty that arise, his motive of action being 'for the welfare of the world'.[1]

From the above considerations it is easy to account for the statement that there arises the perception or understanding (*bodha*) of the 'howness' (*kathantā*) of the course of births (*janman*).[2] The common word for rebirth or reincarnation is *punarjanman*, *punar* meaning 'again'. This yogi has understood the theory very well. He can judge why certain conditions and happenings come to people, and therefore he has the wisdom to see how they should be dealt with to fill up the deficiencies of character of the people involved in them, and when he attains the higher vision or the intuitive or direct perception of the mind, on account of his detachment from particular things, he will positively see the course of past births – that is the meaning.

6. The results of bodily cleanliness are given as 'protectiveness of the body' and 'detachment from others'.

The first part of this explanation of results has been the cause of much conflict of opinion among the commentators. One school of thought takes the word *jugupsā* to mean protectiveness, and another loathing. This is one of those words, rare in Sanskrit, which can have two or more quite different meanings. I have preferred protectiveness for the reason

1. *Bhagavad Gītā*, iii, 20, 25.　　2. *Yoga Sūtras*, ii, 39.

that it accords with common sense and with intelligent practice. It would be strange indeed that dislike of the body should arise from a habit of cleanliness. Desire to protect it from dirt and from 'bad living magnetism' is much more likely. Besides, loathing of anything is as much disapproved in yoga theory as infatuation. The fact that some fanatics despise the body only indicates their own admission of its unnaturalness and the grip which that idea has upon them.

For the sake of cleanliness, and also for the sake of 'psychic cleanliness', the Hindus do not in general approve of bodily contacts. An example is their greeting on meeting one another. The open hands are placed together, palm to palm and fingers to fingers, and held vertically in front of the chest for a moment. This is preferred to the handclasp, which anyhow was originally a way of ensuring the absence of weapons. Other evidence of their carefulness in this matter is the dislike of the upper classes for smoking, with the exception of some who have been influenced by Western customs. One man gave me his reasons: 'I dislike very much the idea of taking into my lungs smoke which has been in other people's mouths and is saturated with their saliva.'

So there is really no justification for the translation of the aphorism as 'loathing for one's own members, and non-intercourse with others'. Besides the reasons already given, this does not fit in very well with the interest in excellence of the body shown in some other aphorisms already quoted, and the general idea that attachment and aversion are both emotions to be overcome. In practice I have found that the great number of people who do yoga meditations every morning are very scrupulous about taking the morning bath and using clean clothing. Dirtiness among Indians is nearly always due to poverty and inconvenience in the water supply.

Patanjali has another aphorism which has been alluded to in this connexion: 'Everything is painful to the discriminating person', or in another translation, 'To the enlightened all is misery'.[1] To the enlightened (*vivekin*), of course. Nothing in the world will compare with nirvāna, and all of us find the limitations of the body irksome, if we think of them. Buddha also laid it down as the first of his 'four noble truths' that all here is sorrow. Every one of our pleasures is tinctured with it. But that did not constitute a condemnation of the world, for in his second noble truth he said, 'Because of your desires.' It was a slap in the face for the common human being. It was the answer to the question why everything was sorrow: 'It is your own fault.' We may add: 'Not the world's fault.' More, there was the implication that as the trouble lay with the individual he could remove it, as shown by the third noble truth, 'Sorrow's ceasing, by the ceasing of your desires'. And finally, the way to this cessation, the fourth noble truth, which was not any sort of suicide, not any shrinking from the world and life, but 'The noble Eight-fold Path' of:

(1) Correct understanding, views, outlook, appraisal, judgement.
(2) Correct aims, motives, plans, decision.
(3) Correct use of speech.
(4) Correct behaviour, conduct, actions.
(5) Correct mode of livelihood.
(6) Correct effort – some good work.
(7) Correct intellectual activity – some study.
(8) Correct contemplation.

Taking care of the body may be regarded as part of this path, for the body is needed for the treading of it. It is only an instrument, we know, and not the perfect man, but it is a means to that end. It is a box of tools to be kept clean, not a bag of filth. Its marvellous excretory and eliminative system illustrates how hard it works to get rid of what we put into it, and the residue of waste resulting from its work for us.

The second result of cleanliness had reference to pure thoughts and words:

From mind-cleanliness come high-mindedness, concentration, mastery of the senses, and fitness for the vision of the Self (*ātma-darshana*).[2]

1. *ibid.*, ii, 15.   2. *ibid.*, ii, 41.

7. The result of Contentment is 'Obtaining of the highest form of pleasure'.[1] This might easily be taken to mean that contentment itself constitutes the greatest pleasure, but that is not what is intended. As all these 'ten commandments' of yoga are virtues for daily living, so also are the results of those concerned with daily living – the efforts and merits are of this world; so also are the rewards. The next likely error to avoid is to think that this contentment implies negative acceptance of things as they are. Yet it does imply the acceptance of things and people as they are and for what they are, namely, materials for living, that is, for the application of our powers of mind and heart – our will, love, and thought.

Contentment is the basis or springboard for fuller living. We have to review every now and then our available materials, our tools, and our intentions. One thing is clear: if there is to be any decided success on the path of yoga – there must be no more complaints, no whining, no grousing, not even any wishing. We need all our powers for the work in hand, whereas every wish is a cultivation of weakness, an announcement to ourselves of our inability to live realistically. Decisions governing actions there will be. By making decisions the will grows; by allowing love to play its part in them our expansion of living and consciousness have their growth, and by the use of thought the power of our thought grows.

As these grow they play a larger and larger part in the moulding of our circumstances and the making of our environment. What is the enhancement of life and consciousness but an increase in our capacity for enjoyment? Contentment paves the way for the three kinds of positive living which constitute the three rules for daily living next to be described – the last three of the 'ten commandments' of the yoga. In the meantime, the acceptance of things and people as they are, with glad acceptance, not wishing them to be different, will enable the yogi to live among them without antagonism, and to derive the maximum pleasure from each

1. *ibid.*, ii, 42.

moment's opportunity. 'We used to live in a big house; now we have to put up with a little one'; 'We used to be well-to-do and to count socially, but now we are poor and despised'; 'These fruits are not as good as those we had in Jamaica five years ago'; 'This film show is no good, does not compare with ...'. Such are the attitudes to avoid, by which we may cause the good and the best to be our undoing, as far as pleasure is concerned.

There is a question whether contentment can be put on like a garment. It can. First it may come from the understanding of life, a proper philosophy which tells us that all things are possible for us in rotation but not all at once, and that each thing has great value for the inner man. Secondly, when it has been known and felt – for it is a discovery still to be made by most people – the mood of the mind can be commanded. Now and then, when you find the discontent, you can command yourself to enjoy, with full attention to what you are doing. Even the enemy is then seen, and felt, as a friend, and we approach the yogic realization that we can be at peace with the world even when the world is not at peace with us.

8. From strict government of the body, amounting even to austerity (tapas), comes excellence of the bodily powers and senses. There is to be no mere indulgence; if certain foods are believed to be best for your body you take them; if they are not good you avoid them. Proper food, exercise, rest, recreation – and all in their proper measure.

It is doubtful whether the word 'austerity' is a satisfactory translation of tapas. Body-conditioning describes the aim. The word tapas comes from a verbal root which means 'to heat', so perhaps our word 'ardour' – applied to bodily living – would be good. Determination to live up to one's knowledge of what is best is implied. Definitely it is the use of will-power in this practical field. We shall find, as we proceed in the study of yoga, that several physical practices are recommended for the welfare of the body and for improvements in its functioning. They include chiefly exercises for purification, breathing, and posture. Those are not, however, included in the term *tapas*, which has to do with strictness in daily life.

9. From study of what really concerns us comes 'connexion with the desired divinity'. There we have indeed to pause and think, to understand the yoga point of view. It is universally accepted in India that we are very dependent beings. That the essential Self is eternal, pure, happy, and free is accepted, and to realize or know that truth by direct experience is the aim of yoga, as has been shown in our previous chapter; but in all matters pertaining to body and mind we are definitely very dependent beings. We need help or food in every part of our being – the 'bread from heaven' as well as the bread of earth. This dependence is the outcome of our collective living, in which each one benefits by association with many, and each one is expected to contribute to this mutual benefit, according to his power.

This concept is extended into the field of knowledge. The study of the great thoughts of others helps us in our understanding. The name for this ninth virtue indicates this. It is *swa* (own) *adhyāya* (study), or study of one's own nature and proper living. In addition, in some way God (*Īshwara*) is the teacher of us all, and all those men of the past who have achieved their independence or divinity are part of That. The laws are not purely external to us. We are learning the inner laws of our being as well as the laws of nature. The *gurus* of the past have left their knowledge 'in the atmosphere' – not the ultimate knowledge, of course, which can never be brought down or represented. There is much that exists above us in Nature, as well as below, and that companionship can be brought within our scope. We can eat of that bread of life, which is there for us when we reach up to it, and may appear in our lives as intuition, and, with some who anthropomorphize their experiences, as from angels or divine beings, who belong to the region of Law and can represent and teach it. Sincere study, the aphorism teaches, will lead to and enhance our contact with this desired 'divinity'.

10. Finally, the reward of attentiveness to God is the power of contemplation or success in contemplation

(*samādhi*). The world might be fantastic and unbelievable, but it is not. It also might be fantastic and unreliable with regard to goodness, but it is not. Constantly the devotional yogi sees more and more, in many of the experiences of life, that it is not, and even how it is not. There is therefore gratitude – that the Laws are sane and good and that we are at all times enveloped in that sanity and goodness. To be aware of this sanity and goodness and to be grateful for it is a sort of contemplation or poise of the heart and mind, which passes from gratitude to worship. Worship is thus our highest function, the 'flowering and completion of human culture', as Emerson called it. It is contemplation of the absolute presence of the Divine, and naturally its function is the perfection of itself.

Although the eight steps of yoga proceed next to posture, then to breathing, then on to control of the senses, and only in the sixth, seventh, and eighth stages deal with concentration, meditation, and contemplation, which are the inner or mental steps, we will now proceed in our next chapter to study the Intellectual steps, and afterwards take up posture, etc., to see how they support the main purpose.

CHAPTER 4

YOGA AND THE INTELLECT

IT is in the last three of the eight limbs of yoga presented in the *Yoga Sūtras* that we find the training and use of the mind. In this there are three clearly defined stages. These three may be translated as:

> Concentration (*dhāranā*)
> Meditation (*dhyāna*)
> Contemplation (*samādhi*)

In the first of these there is the application of the mind's attention to a particular thing or idea, without wandering away from it. This non-wandering constitutes what is called control (*nirodha*).

In the second of the three, namely meditation, there is a play of thought upon the object. While this is going on the concentration is still in operation, but the play of thought goes on with reference to the object of attention without passing away to other things. Thus, for example, if the object is a flower there will be every possible thought about the flower. Usually in looking at things we are content to note a few outstanding features and the same is true also in our thinking about them, but in meditation there should be complete thinking, if possible.

A and B were at a party last night. Today A says to B, 'Do you remember Mrs Whelkson, who was there?' B replies, 'Yes, I remember her very clearly. She was the lady with the big nose.' A then asks, 'What was the colour of her eyes and her hair and dress?' B can only reply that he has not even the foggiest notion.

The usual thinking of most people is based upon data almost as bad as this. In matters philosophical or devotional, with which yoga is very much concerned, this will not do.

Hence the need for the three processes already named, which are thus described in the aphorisms:

The binding of the mind (*chitta*) to one place is concentration (*dhāranā*).

Continuity of ideation there is meditation (*dhyāna*).

The same, but with the shining of the mere object, as though with a voidness of one's own nature, is contemplation (*samādhi*).[1]

In the last of the three the reader may recognize the chief characteristic of ecstasy or rapture. In that one forgets oneself, is taken out of oneself, yet is intensely conscious. The quality of consciousness is, in fact, at its best. This is not an emotional state, but an operation of seeing or knowing, in which there is nothing partial and nothing brought to the picture from memory, or from the past, to colour the present experience with any comparison or classification. If you were looking at a picture, and saying, 'How nice it is. See this group of trees here, and that little stream there, and that light on the hillside ...', you would be experiencing the delight of meditative examination, which would gradually build the picture into one unit, as you grasped these various interesting items clearly and then combined them into one and discovered the unity of the whole. But if you 'took in' the whole picture at once, missing nothing, not flitting among the parts from one to another, you would undergo ecstatic discovery and experience of the unity. For this, the picture must of course be good; that is, there must be no slightest mark on the canvas which is not necessary, just as, for example, in an excellent human body all the parts must be there, but there must be no redundancy, such as an extra thumb growing on the side of the proper one.

Such pictures are possible when there is an inspiration representing one idea in which all the components are necessary and none in conflict. Such pictures, if landscapes, will have their origin in a peaceful scene, in which the elements do not molest one another – sea is sea, mountain mountain, cloud cloud, and sky sky – and yet they set one another off; indeed, the harmony of Nature discovered by

1. *Yoga Sūtras*, iii, 1–3.

the scientist tells us that these are necessary to one another. As long as you are seeing the harmonies you are *thinking*, or, if it is systematic, you are *meditating*, but if you are seeing it all and seeing it *whole* you are no longer thinking, but *knowing*, even if knowing by seeing.

Knowing is not thinking. Knowing begins when thinking ceases, having finished its work. Every new knowing is a joy, for it is a new experience of unity – something perfectly attuned and non-conflicting in Nature has conveyed its lesson, nay, has entered and enriched the being of the consciousness, just as edibles and air enter the body and become part of it. Every idea is a unit, however many connected thoughts may be associated within it.

Every new experience of knowledge – more properly described as an act of knowledge – will in due course become a mere part of a still greater or more inclusive vision. All new thinking or meditation leads to this until the very *summum genus* of knowing is reached – that One to realize which is the supreme aim of the yogi. In successive meditations one reviews the old ground, and in so doing finds that new thoughts arise. In this way there is repetition with newness.

The word *samādhi* not only names the contemplation of a unity but also describes it. In common use the word means agreement. In its use in the mind it implies a complete absence of any conflict of ideas. It arises when the process of meditation on any subject reaches its end, having completely coordinated all the contents of the mind which have relation to that subject, including every memory that can be recalled and every thought that can be thought with respect to the subject or object. When that meditation has been done the idea is one organic unit, and it stands in one piece, just as when we say 'man' it is one idea, including all the various parts. It is not a combination but an integration of particulars. And those parts and particulars then take their character from the Whole or One, just as fingers are fingers only because they are part of the hand. *Samādhi* is seeing that unity, whether in a man or other object, or a picture or a piece of music. That is why in a good picture there must not be one unnecessary stroke, and in a good piece of music not one unnecessary note.[1]

It is not to be supposed that every practice or act of meditation or contemplation must have as its object something very large. It should deal only with the whole of the thing prescribed, and even then only what concerns the *one idea* which is the object of meditation. The aesthetic idea of a tree does not include the roots. The aesthetic idea of the human body does not include the internal organs. This is where *wisdom* comes in – the knowledge of what is good to know. The fox going out for food in the evening needs to know only what it needs to know, but it certainly does need to know that. The same applies to man, and to the meditator.

From all these considerations it will be seen that concentration, meditation, and contemplation form a connected series. Before you meditate you choose your subject or object of meditation, and there is then an act of will in which you tell your mind to keep to that subject and not to wander away from it.

This concentration on the chosen subject then goes on by itself, and you need not think of it. If you have decided to walk in a certain direction the legs go on walking; you need not think of this act of will at every step. An act of will goes on operating until another act of will changes it. Similarly, the act of concentration is still there while the meditation is going on, though it has been forgotten – 'subconscious' or 'unconscious' is the new word for this, though really it is now a habit, an act of the mind lapsed into inert form or motion.

It is to be remembered, of course, when studying these three successive operations of the mind, that meditation and contemplation are not states of mind but *functionings* of mind. They are something you are *doing*. The man is not 'in medi-

1. The main part of the word *samādhi* is *dhi* (idea), which is found also in the word '*dhyāna*'. The prefix *sam* indicates union or togetherness and with *ā* there is a strengthening of the idea of coming together.

tation'; he is meditating. The well-known fact that the mind improves or grows by exercise applies here. In the early days of the practice of meditation the student often finds his mind very dull. It does not bring forth many thoughts. But as the practice proceeds it will be found that the mind becomes active and brings forth a veritable fountain of thoughts. Even so, on a given subject, or object of thought, the fountain will come to the end of its resources. If then the intention (the will, the concentration) still goes on (now being in a void of thinking) there will be intuition or illumination. Something quite new, not seen or thought of before, will arise. It will at the same time bring delight, for there is an enrichment of consciousness.

It is not that one's consciousness is enriched by a new thought, or enhanced by an accumulation of thoughts (like the stamp collection of a philatelist). It is rather an awakening or a growth of conscious being and power. All the objects of perception and thought are thus very much like a little girl's doll. The doll does not do anything; the child does everything. The child awakens and enhances its own being. The doll only provides a ground for the concentration and meditation, which the little girl is unconsciously doing when she plays with it. Her mother would be far from pleased if she saw that the girl was only accumulating dolls, and not growing into a woman.

It is not desirable that the girl when playing with the doll should think of this process or its results. She should not be saying to herself, 'I am playing with this doll in order to grow into a mother.' What conception of mother-love can the child have before it is developed? The child is having pleasure only, but that prepares the ground for the awakening of love. Prior to that awakening, the child's thought, if so directed, could only lead to a wrong picture – quite likely to egotism and self-satisfaction, of which mother-love is quite the reverse.

The good teacher of meditation tells the student not to think of the results of his practices. In entering upon a meditation he *must not* predetermine the results, for the reason that he is going to arrive at something which he does not previously know. These meditations must be undertaken *without desire*, if one would have the newness of life. This is the setting aside of 'the *old* man' and the opening of the door to 'newness of life'.

There is not in this advice to meditate the assumption that the aspirant is aiming at great things. The trouble with us is that we do not know anything well, or well enough, or we are far from knowing it as it is. What do we know, for example, of strength, or love, or courage, or the wing of a butterfly? The crudity of the average mind is almost incredible. 'Meditate on the strength of the elephant,' says the yogi, and then you will get a better conception of strength – not a definition of strength, but an experience of strength in the mind. All things have qualities. To see those qualities well is to have them in the mind. The relaxedness and the alertness of the cat can be ours not by mental formulation and definition, but by contemplation. All things are qualities, and we can be one with a group of those, in one act of direct perception.

The Practice of Meditation. The teacher of concentration often tells his students simply to go on trying to keep the attention upon one thing, and bring it back whenever it wanders, until at last it obeys, like a 'broken-in' horse, and concentration then becomes a habit. This is not the best way; it lacks psychological subtlety.

Let it be noticed, first of all, that the mind has a habit of drifting – picture follows picture on a line of least resistance, or a line of habit, and this is mostly habit of the emotions, of desires and aversions born of past pleasures and pains. Thus if one says 'cow', the succession of so-called thoughts may be 'milk – baby – cot – furniture store – Stenton's – San Francisco – Golden Gate Bridge – iron-foundry – fire – forest fire-fleeing animals – running – Olympic games –' and so on, over the hills and far away.

The second thing to notice is that we have the power to stop this flow, and often do so. For example, in the series given, we might stop at the bridge and begin to go over the picture of the bridge. We might even start wondering about its material, its design, and indeed many things. The exercise of this power is concentration.

In concentration the same picture is attended to in successive moments. Some people ensure this by the repetition of a word. But when the power of concentration is established there should be no need of such repetition. It should be enough that you have decided to attend to the idea of the bridge. Further, such attention may be actual. Disregarding for the time being all the rest of the scenery, you may decide to look at the bridge more carefully than before. From this comes the term concentration. You are bringing your diffused attention to a focus on a comparatively small thing. Then, of course, you will see it better than ever you did before. All the same, actual visualization in meditation is not necessary; people differ very much in this respect, and it is not important.

This can be done with small things also, such as a bit of colour or a sound, by giving exclusive attention to it. Near me on the table there is a kitchen towel with a pattern of red squares, or rather with red lines leaving white squares. That red colour is pleasing, and as I attend to it closely I find that I see the redness of the red better than I have seen red before. The same would also apply to notes on the musical scale. If we have not acquired some precision in observing these or hearing them carefully at some time in the past there will surely be some deficiency in our ability to appreciate music, and probably we shall like only that 'music' which is thrust at us blaringly and crudely – something that compels our attention. Some things compel our attention, some attract it, but in yoga we aim to have voluntary attention, so that we may properly awaken or grow, and properly reproduce things on the screen of imagination for the purposes of thought.

Another important thing to notice is that for concentration you do not need force or tension. Calm looking is best. It is just bad habit which makes us think that intensity helps. In practice, it is found to be quite the reverse. Attention without tension is best for success in concentration, and best for the welfare of the body, which suffers from the strain of the tension, whereas it would gain by being quiet.

With these precautions we may now turn to the scientific practice of concentration:

Choose your subject for practice – say, a cow. Then think of everything that you can concerning the cow, without losing sight of the cow. Thus you may review its parts – horns, hoofs, tail, milk, etc.; its qualities – placidity, timidity, colour, weight, etc.; its characteristics as an animal in comparison with other animals; and 'cows I have known'. Do not stop until you have thought of all the items you can. If necessary continue the same subject through several sittings.

I have recommended beginners to practise at first with the aid of a sheet of paper, instead of merely trying to do it in mind. Place a large sheet of paper on the table; write the word cow in the middle of it; surround that by a circle, and draw projecting arrows all round it, thus:

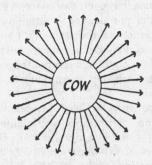

Look at the word 'cow'; close the eyes and think of it; note the first thought that comes into your mind, say, milk; open your eyes and write the word 'milk' at the end of one of the arrows. Do not think about milk (which would lead you away to cats or babies or the Milky Way), but slide your eye back to the cow at the centre.

Close the eyes, and wait for another word to come up, say, 'tufted tail'; open the eyes and write 'tufted tail'. Do not think about a tail, but return to the centre, as before. Continue. You may get twenty or thirty arrow-words. Continue. There will be some waiting and searching, but continue. You may get forty or fifty words. Continue; and do not give up until at least five minutes after no more words come.

In this way you acquire concentration without thinking about concentration. After several practices your mind learns to keep to a subject when previously directed to do so, instead of wandering and dissipating its energies. There arises a *mood of return* to the centre. After a little while you can put this mood on like a garment. You have found the feel of it, and now a small act of will sets it in operation, just as you walk and go somewhere definite as the result of a small act of will. You do not need to think of concentration, but can swing your mind round to things and thoughts, or from one to another, with great and calm definiteness. You can then use this for all kinds of mental work – reading, studying, writing, lecturing, teaching, etc.

In yoga practice, however, this concentration is used as a step to the further practices of meditation and contemplation. These are functions, something that you do, not static conditions and states. Even contemplation (*samādhi*) is something that you *do*, though it is not thinking, and you do not think about it when you are doing it, once you have acquired it.

In the practice with the sheet of paper, let us notice the difference between concentration and meditation. After you have completed your concentration you possess a sheet of paper with many arrow-words on it. For the elementary exercises of meditation lay this completed sheet on the table, note the first arrow-word, for example, milk. Do not forget it or put it out of mind, as you did in the elementary concentration practice, but slide your eye back to the cow, carrying the idea of milk with you, and then *think*. Think all you can about the relations between the milk and the cow. When this is finished (and only you can judge as to when this is, but let the judgement not be motivated by impatience or the desire to get it done and done with), turn to the next arrow-word – the tufted tail – and deal with it in the same manner. And so on.

This will lead on to contemplation. Quite often people fall into contemplation without thinking of it, until – this is important – they find themselves coming out of it, much to their surprise. They have the memory of the enjoyment of consciousness in the now terminated act of contemplation. As they look back upon it they realize that they were they without thinking of themselves, but only contemplating the object. Out of it they come, back into their meditative mood, bringing something new back with them – some thought that they did not think in their meditation. It is an intuition, an item of knowing, or something that illumines the entire field, the whole subject, every part of it. Still more: after a while they come to know what contemplation *feels like*, and then can switch into it, through an act of concentration and meditation that seems to take no time. It is another mood, known only by experience, and then as a power of the mind.

Have we any examples in common life of occurrences or acts presaging this ability? Yes, we often 'lose ourselves'. We peep into someone's office or study, and tip-toe away, whispering to our companions, 'He is lost in thought.' I knew a man who used to lecture frequently, on subjects requiring much thought. He told me that he had acquired the power to put himself out of mind – completely forget himself – at the commencement of a lecture, and look mentally at his subject-matter like a map on which he was following a route, while the spoken words flowed in complete obedience to the successive ideas which were being looked at. He told me that he would become aware of himself perhaps once or twice during the lecture, and at the end of it, as he sat down, he would find himself surprised that it was he who had given the lecture. Yet he fully remembered everything; only 'himself' (the common idea or picture of self) being absent.

It is incredible to those who have not had the experience that man can thus enjoy life beyond mind. To make a comparison, it is incredible to the body that the mind can manipulate inside itself (in imagination) thousands of facts, and similarly it is incredible to the mind-self (pictured, as it is, as one of those facts) that consciousness can be enjoyed without it. The truth is that 'I' is not then eliminated, but is revealed to itself as no object. That is what our 'I' always is, but the mind clothes it in thought, and looks at it from the outside.

There are certain conditions which go against this attainment. In his *Vedanta Sāra* (Essence of Vedanta), Sadānanda Swāmī has called them the four enemies of *samādhi*: a sleepy heart, attachment to anything but Brahman, human passions, and a confused mind.

One must not here, in the chapter on mind-process, go into the full discussion of Self or I.

In the standard descriptions of *samādhi*, or contemplation, two kinds are usually mentioned, and described as:

(1) with consciousness of an object (*samprajnāta*), and
(2) without consciousness of an object (*asamprajnāta*).

The former of these two is an earlier stage of attainment than the latter. Still, it is not only a step on the way to the latter. It is definitely a platform of conscious living, and has a definite ability of its own. While the latter is concerned with meditation about what is beyond subject and object, the former is concerned with things known in the world. In the course of this perceptive form of meditation and *samādhi* there are two stages:

(*a*) Inspectional (*vitarka*), and
(*b*) Investigational (*vichāra*).

The inspectional is concerned with objective things as known in time and space, and therefore often described as dense or gross. The object of this state is to get a clear image in consciousness of the object chosen for meditation at any given time.

The investigational is intended to find out the subtle characters or abstract natures of such things, that is, the characteristics and qualities of them which are not visible to the senses. This requires much thought about categories or classes of the objects, and their constants behind time and space. Let us take as our example the notion of a cow. In the *vitarka* stage we shall observe what it is, what it has, and what it does in fact. These are being, doing, and having at the concrete level. In the *vichāra* stage we shall be concerned with the cow as cow and as such something beyond time and space, which is the same in all circumstances and at all times, and is always in the same manner causative in its relation to other beings and objects. The particular objective cow can be regarded as expressive of a subtle reality which it embodies. The subtle is thus something of the nature of mind. Thinking is required to get at these abstracts and to see that they are realities and are the powers in the world, or the axes of all growth.

Instead of an object, like the cow, one may consider the senses of hearing, feeling or touching, seeing, tasting, and smelling. These are not considered to be *derived* from objects (as though salt had a certain taste and sugar a certain taste; which they have not, for sugar is not sweet to itself) but are deep-seated axes of the growth of forms and are responsible for the relations of selves to things, including their bodies and minds. As such they are realities to be known by much thinking (*vichāra*). Only their effects at the gross (*sthūla*) level are matters for inspection by the senses. These subtle objects of enquiry go on from depth to depth, even as far as the indefinable reality which we call the undifferentiated manifest reality (*prakriti*). The aphorism states this in the following terms: 'The domain of the subtle ends only at the indefinable'.[1]

This can be understood by remembering that the ultimate class or ultimate substance in this case cannot be known in terms of its presentations, which limit it by particularity, and so do not represent it.

In this philosophy – or science – both things and mind are material (*prakriti*), though the first are gross and the latter subtle, though the first have form and the latter is formless, though the first are of space (have spatial dimensions or extensity, or exist as space-process), and the latter is not of

1. *ibid.*, i, 45.

space (has no extensity) but exists as a time-process. Therefore meditations can go to the indefinable *summum genus*,
or ultimate class, and there they must stop, because
there is nothing thinkable about, as there are no
characteristics.

We have now to understand that both the inspectional
and investigational kinds of meditation and contemplation
are dealing with something of the world (of the object-side
or of the mind-side of it), and they are therefore operating
within the field of matter (*prakriti*). As such their results are
also within that field. On this account they are described as
'with seed' (*sabija*). If the meditation and contemplation are
on a cow the resulting intuition will be something about a
cow.

Another point to be noted is that each of the two forms
of materially-conscious (*samprajñāta*) meditation and contemplation has two stages. Thus there are:

    (*a*) The inspectional (*savitarka*) and the
    (*b*) Non-inspectional (*nirvitarka*).

Similarly, there are:

    (*a*) The Investigational (*savichāra*) and the
    (*b*) Non-investigational (*nirvichāra*).

When the inspectional observation of the cow is complete,
one can pause there and contemplate it, as then known
(*savitarka*), or one can try to get something more by an
intent contemplation of feeling (love or rapport, great
interest) or by will (*nirvitarka*). There is an argument, as it
were, about words, meaning, and knowledge.

In this condition, when the seed has germinated and some
intuition has come, one is ready for the investigational
practice and, in due course, the non-investigational. There
is, however, no hard and fast rule in this matter. The
student must follow his inclinations, unless he has the
privilege of being the pupil of a teacher (*guru*) who can
unerringly see all his thoughts. Even then, the teacher
usually leaves him mostly to self-devised efforts, knowing
that the decisions thus involved are a part – the most important part – of the training.

When the intuition has come, in any degree, there is a sense of delight which sustains the condition. This is *ānanda* and is an experience of the state of mind in connexion with the object. And next comes sense of being, not merely of knowing but of being the knower (*asmitā*), a conscious ability of self-government, over which one's thoughts and feelings cannot prevail. This is coming near the mountain top or peak (*kūtastha*). We could call them respectively the enjoyment of knowing and the enjoyment of the sense of power of knowing, or self-enhancement.

In the investigational and non-investigational meditation and contemplation the seed (*bīja*) will lead to some intuition with respect to the subtle matters under consideration, and to great growth of the mind, even to its complete maturity.

Beyond these four stages there is the contemplation without the idea of subject and object, of the seer and the seen (*asamprajnāta samādhi*). In this the student has to become conscious of the spirit (*purusha*). Before this he has been concerned with observing the world or the mind, or both. It becomes necessary to realize that the body is not conscious, but we are conscious of the body, also that the mind is not conscious but we are conscious of the mind. A first glimpse of this can be gained from the following occurrence:

One day a teacher of meditation (*guru*) told one of his pupils to walk to the far end of the room and back and sit down. Then he asked:

'What were you doing just now? Were you walking?'

The pupil went over his action mentally, and observed everything that he had done, and then replied:

'I was not walking. I was watching the body walk.'

Next the teacher held up a flower and asked him to meditate upon it for a few minutes. After this had been done the teacher questioned:

'What were you doing just now? Were you meditating?'

After due observation and reflection the pupil answered:

'I was not meditating. I was watching the mind meditate.'

In this manner the pupil acquired a sudden discrimination between the self and the mind. He had a momentary release from the thought of himself as mind.

Now he became fit for the practice of the super-conscious (*asamprajnāta*) or seedless (*nirbīja*) *samādhi*. He would now set his mind to think of the unthinkable – God; the Absolute; Consciousness; Self; Reality. Can he think of what is beyond matter and its varieties, beyond mind and its categories or classes? The mind says, 'No'; yet he has had the experience in the moment of discrimination (*viveka*).

The pupil did not know it before, but he has had the experience. He will now set himself the seemingly impossible task. He will tell his mind to think on God, Truth, Reality, Self, Consciousness, the Absolute.... There is no gas for this ballooning; nothing on earth or in the mind can help him. He must make no comparisons or contrasts, no definitions, no categories. He must use his own jet-power to ride over all these things. In his practice he can use words (1) to keep other thoughts out of the picture, and (2) to act as boats for the voyage of discovery. These are not words of definition, but words of discovery.

He will find that he has to perform this feat by an act (or acts) of being. He will know the being, because the being has its own knowing, which is direct, without any intermediate or mediating thing or thought. This act of being is sustained by his will. He has set his face towards the *fulfilment* of the will. After all, all his doing and having in the past has only been operated to serve his experience of being. We do not fundamentally want *to have* and *to do;* we only want *to be*, and we use the having and doing for that purpose. Further, our will to be is not content with anything; it seeks its goal beyond the irksome limits of having and doing. Man will not be really happy until he is consciously one with God, and shares the freedom of that one Reality.

There in the will is indeed another seed, but it is the seed not of anything in the world or in the mind, but of the Beyond which alone accounts for the 'here'. The will never changes; it always points to that true North. The mind is of the mud of earth, except in this one fact. Therein is that spark of original power and being, even in the midst of the mind and the body. Man cannot master other things, because all have the right to master themselves; but man can master himself and be without fear. He can learn that all things serve him and he them, and that nothing in his life happens contrary to his will, which is so little known by the rest of his mind, which yet can come to know and thus enter that glorious service, and will come to know this through the *asamprajñāta samādhi*. 'Man is the mirror of the universe', it has been said. Yes, and in this point of joyous vision and service the mirror of God and his freedom, reality, truth, self, and all. Thus he will find God here, even in the mind, and be able to say from experience, 'He who cannot find God here cannot find him anywhere'.

In some of the preceding paragraphs I have mentioned meditation and contemplation together. The reason for this is that concentration, meditation, and contemplation form a sequence, always together. The act or practice begins with concentration, which then continues inside or behind the meditation. It goes on with meditation and then continues in or behind the contemplation, which remains within its scope.

Still, nothing goes on forever, and the upward way is like a stair, not an inclined plane. Each stair or platform prepares for the next. In childhood we develop mostly our bodies and senses. Later, when these are mature and have practically stopped growing we develop especially our emotions. Later still, our thoughts, and at last some synthetic wisdom. Therein lies the doctrine of the archetypes. It would not do for our bodies to grow a hundred feet tall; the leverages would be wrong, say the biologists. Yet there is some degree that can be called perfect body. When it reaches that, it stops. So also with emotions and mind. The archetype is not a blueprint, a prototype, but a limit. It is not perfection in the abstract.

We can have perfect dog, perfect cat, perfect cow, and then if the life is to go on, it must inhabit something else. So, when the mind is matured by experience or meditation, it is logical and natural that something new should manifest, or that a spark of newness which was always there should now become a flame which, with its light and power, will create and govern the new scene.

It is very important that the student should not feel discouraged. For one thing, he should remember that whatever meditation is done in periods allotted to it, or in spare minutes of opportunity, leaves its permanent gain. It is like physical exercise in this respect; ten minutes in the morning will result in better health and strength all day.

It will help if the student remembers that meditation is not a condition in which one is, but is a function which one is performing. Compare it with walking; walking is not a condition which you are in, but is a function you are performing. The same applies also to such matters as breathing and digesting, but in this case the function has become a habit or has been handed over to the physical dynamic habit mechanism.

This remark applies to all the three 'inner' limbs (*angas*) of yoga, named concentration (*dhāranā*), meditation (*dhyāna*), and contemplation (*samādhi*), which are numbers 6, 7, and 8 in the series of eight limbs. All the 'limbs' are something that you *do*, not something that you *are*. Because these three are operations of the mind, not of the body, they are described as 'inner limbs' (*antaranga*): 'The three are inner compared with the previous (limbs).'[1]

At this point it is also explained that there is a name for all three, taken together as one operation: 'The three in oneness are poise (*sanyama*).'[2]

---

1. *ibid.*, iii, 7.
2. *ibid.*, iii, 4. The word *sanyama* has been translated by some as 'restraint', so it becomes necessary for me to explain my translation of it as poise. If the word *yama* means to restrain or hold back, as it does in the five Abstentions, and the same with *ni* in *niyama* means to hold steady (the verb *niyam* is, in fact, used for the binding up of the long hair), the *sanyama* (the prefix *san* meaning 'together') can easily be understood as 'holding together'. Such an idea is not to be confused with checking, still less with check-mating or stoppage. It does, however, involve a unified poise with reference to the object or idea at a given time under review

The expression 'three in one' indicates that there is a combined action. In practice one begins with concentration (selection of an object), continues with meditation (the fullest possible comprehension of the object), and proceeds to contemplation. The three constitute one operation. To plunge into *samādhi* without previously selecting an object for it is contrary to yoga practice, and could result in a negative condition of mind.

The practice of the mind-poise (*sanyama*) on various selected objects and ideas usually follows a course beginning with simple concrete objects, through complex concrete, simple abstract, complex abstract, the mind processes, and finally the Looker or Self itself (*drashtā, purusha, ātman*). This does not mean that there is to be a laborious sequence every time. After a while concentration becomes very swift – almost momentary – and meditation, or the review of relevancies, almost equally so in a well-known subject. These two stages may be described as respectively 'grip' and 'grasp'.

Many students feel discouraged when they should not. They should not think of results, but do the work when opportunity offers. Celebrated is the case of Arjuna, the disciple of Shrī Krishna in the *Bhagavad Gītā*. The teacher

---

or treatment. It involves, as poise always does, whether in poetry or in the dance, an elimination of irrelevancies. Poise is dynamic – something quite different from pose, which is static.

While on the subject of words in the *Yoga Sūtras* involving the conception of some kind of restraint, it may be well to look at the word 'control' (*nirodha*) as appearing in 'Yoga is control (*nirodha*) of the ideas (*vrittis*; literally "whirlpools") in the mind (*chitta*)' (*Yoga Sūtras*, i, 2). The control of ideas and of idea-impulses involved in this general definition of yoga practice cannot mean mere stoppage or suppression. The definitions of concentration, meditation, and contemplation, already given in this chapter, preclude such a supposition. It is true that thoughts and thinking come to an end and are replaced by direct vision, but this is after meditation, not before it, and the practice involves control, not suppression. Even in *samādhi* there are objects of attention, ending with the mind-poise on discrimination – knowledge (*viveka-khyāti*) which results in the 'looker' (*drashtā*; consciousness) residing in his own state, which is independence (*kaivalya*).

(*guru*) tells the pupil (*shishya*) to make his thinking mind (*manas*) one-pointed (*ekāgra*) and then proceed with his yoga for the purification of himself.[1] 'Whenever,' he says, 'the unsteady mind wanders off, then, having held it firm, let him bring it, controlled, under the Self.'[2]

This was to be done little by little, said Shrī Krishna. Arjuna, however, did not view the task hopefully. He exclaimed, 'The mind (*manas*) is very restless, O Krishna, impetuous, powerful, and firm. I think it is as hard to control as the wind.' The teacher's reply was definite and simple: 'Undoubtedly the mind (*manas*) is restless and hard to control, but it is held by practice (*abhyāsa*) and uncolouredness (*vairāgya*).'[3]

The word 'uncolouredness' may seem rather uncouth, but it well expresses the idea, that one must not let one's emotions be coloured by the various things and ideas which come up. Some have translated this word as 'dispassion', 'indifference', 'non-attachment', etc., but 'uncolouredness' is absolutely literal. The student should notice that anxiety and the feelings of difficulty and of hankering for success are colouring the feelings and the mind, and so he should think of what he is doing, not of results. Then success will accrue.

A further anxiety is next shown by Arjuna. He asks what happens if the aspirant falls away from his purpose, or fails to attain success. Krishna replies that after death he will live in the inner worlds according to his merit, for a long time, and then: 'He who fell from yoga is born (again) in a pure and fortunate house. Or he even comes into a family of wise yogis, though a birth such as this is very hard to obtain in this world. There he obtains the *buddhic* attainments of his previous incarnations, and thence he again strives for full accomplishment.'[4]

A description of the psychic powers available to man, and appearing occasionally among the yogis of India and also quite often in spiritualist and psychic research circles in the West, will find its most appropriate place in this book in

1. *Bhagavad Gītā*, vi, 12.   2. *ibid.*, vi, 26.   3. *ibid.*, vi, 35.
4. *ibid.*, vi, 40–3.

this chapter on 'Yoga and the Intellect'. These powers are considered by their students to be an extension of our perceptions and abilities, and therefore, further adjuncts to the mind. They are not either in the West or in the East regarded as unnatural or supernatural, but rather just further developments of our natural powers, and subject to acceleration of growth by appropriate means. Almost all persons have at some time or other had some small (and sometimes large) indications of such things as telepathy, clairvoyance, and premonition.

One frequently reads about the psychic faculties and powers shown occasionally by yogic experts in India and sometimes in other places. We must distinguish faculties from powers because these phenomena fall into two classes, as indeed our ordinary sense and mind activities also do. Men can perceive things through the sense organs (*jñānendriyas*); they can also act upon the world by the action organs (*karmendriyas*). Indeed it is sometimes said that man lives in 'the ten organs' and the rest of the body is only there to contain them.

The body is thus two-fold with respect to ordinary affairs. The same is true, it is said, with respect to the mind, but the mind is less developed than the body. As it develops more it will use its subtle organs for perceiving, showing the abilities popularly called second sight, psychometry, clairvoyance, clairaudience, etc. Later, when further developed, it is maintained, the mind of each person will show its abilities of action, or what is called direct action of the mind upon matter. The former are called faculties and the latter powers.

In the very extensive and varied yoga literature of India, both classical and modern, there is frequent reference to psychic powers, but not usually – somewhat to the surprise of the Western enquirer – enthusiasm about them. They are regarded as coming by the way, and are not treated as something to be sought for or especially prized. Indeed, the highest authority of all, Patanjali, speaks of the arising of higher senses of hearing, touch, sight, taste, and smell, but immediately adds: 'These powers of the spreading (or outgoing) mind are injurious to contemplation (*samādhi*).'[1]

No objection to them is indicated otherwise than as temptations to linger by the wayside with these new enjoyments, and in fairness to the whole field of study Patanjali in about thirty aphorisms speaks of them and how they are produced. Some of these statements are somewhat obscure at our date, but Patanjali lists a variety of them as resulting from full meditation upon certain things. He also mentions that the powers arise also in other manners than by practise of yoga-meditation, listing them as sometimes occurring from birth, and sometimes produced by means of drugs, incantations (*mantras*), and austerities.[2]

As examples of those produced by full meditation (i.e. concentration, meditation, and contemplation) may be mentioned: knowledge of past and future; understanding of the sounds made by all creatures; knowledge of past lives; knowing what others are thinking; prior knowledge of one's death; the attainment of various kinds of strength; perception of the small, the concealed, and the distant; knowledge of other inhabited regions; knowledge about the stars and their motions; knowledge of the interior of the body; control of hunger and thirst; steadiness; seeing the adepts in one's own interior light; general intuition; understanding of the mind; entering the bodies of others; lightness and levitation; brightness; control of material elements; control of the senses; perfection of the body; quickness of the body, and the well-known set of eight powers beginning with smallness.[3]

Patanjali does not give a list of the eight powers, but it appears frequently and widely in yoga literature. They are:

Minuteness (*animā*). To be as small as an atom, at will.

Expansion (*mahimā*). To increase in size, at will.

Lightness (*laghimā*). Neutralization of gravity, at will.

Reaching (*prāpti*). To obtain anything or to reach any place, at will.

Acquirement (*prākāmya*). To have the fulfilment of any wish, at will.

---

1. *Yoga Sūtras*, iii, 36.   2. *ibid.*, iv, 1.   3. *ibid.*, iii, 16–48.

Lordship (*īshatwā*). Control of the energies of Nature, at will.

Self-control (*vashitwā*). Self-command and freedom from being influenced, at will.

Desire-control (*kāmavasāyita*). The stopping of all desires, at will.

These are interpreted in detail in various ways, subjective and objective, by various yogis, *gurus*, and writers.[1]

Before leaving this topic, it seems desirable to reiterate that the *rāja-yogī* is aiming at the experience of inward illumination beyond all sensation. He is aiming not to be governed by impulses of any kind from outside, however relatively superior. He aims at the mountain-top (*kūtastha*) not to 'rest' on any object (*ālambana*).

A symbol frequently used to emphasize this point is that of the lotus plant. It rises from the mud, grows through the water, and flowers in the air and sunshine. That stem growing upward through the water (when it would be so much easier to lie along the ground at the bottom) knows nothing of the flowering that is to be. Yet it responds to an *inner* impulse. So the *rāja-yogī* obeys an inner impulse, not presuming to state to himself what the flowering will be like. The simile of the grub and the butterfly is also used to illustrate the aim of the *rāja-yogī*. The seeker of psychic powers, on the other hand, is still under the fascination of known things, and is only asking for them to be enhanced. As St Paul puts it, the proper aim is newness of life and the setting aside of the *old* man.

1. The lists differ. In my *Yoga Dictionary* I have given heaviness (*garimā*) instead of desire-control, but here I have allowed heaviness to be assumed along with lightness. In my *Glorious Presence* I have simplified them into unlimited smallness, largeness, lightness, heaviness, vision, movement, creativeness, and control.

CHAPTER 5

THE BREATHING PRACTICES
OF YOGA

IN the foregoing chapters we have considered what may be called the spiritual or ultimate aim of yoga, then the ethical and moral principles, and then the intellectual. We come now to study the teachings of yoga concerning the body.

These are given in Patanjali's list as of three kinds – the limbs (*angas*) of yoga dealing with (*a*) posture (*āsana*), (*b*) with breathing (*prānāyāma*), and (*c*) with control of the senses (*pratyāhāra*).

The practice of *prānāyāma* can be described as voluntary control of inbreathing, outbreathing, and holding the breath. This is done chiefly for the setting up of a new condition of breathing intended to become habitual after sufficient voluntary practice. In this connexion it is found that the transition from effort to habit is accompanied by a feeling in the mind (which we may call a mood), growing and becoming definite in the course of the process, whereby later on at any time when one finds that the breathing has reverted to a bad or undesired habit one may remember the feel of the mood, and with an almost imperceptible act of will, re-establish the new habit.

The growth of this 'mood' implies that while the outer actions are being practised the inner 'power' is being cultivated. This is quite analogous to what takes place when a swimmer approaches the water; by a very slight remembering of the mood of the mind during swimming he instantly adapts a complex system of physical reflexes to the act of swimming. There is a story about a lady who fell off a pleasure steamer. She was a good swimmer, but on this occasion she thrashed about and showed every sign of being about to drown until suddenly she became quite calm and was seen to be swimming steadily towards the boat. On being asked afterwards, she explained that she was confused and did not know what had happened until suddenly she regained her wits and exclaimed to herself, 'Why! I am in the water,' and then she swam.

A second purpose of the practice of *prāṇāyāma* is to develop a few techniques which may be used (and also may become temporary habits connected with moods) on special occasions. Just as our breathing changes during exertion, so it can change when there is a fall or rise of temperature affecting the body, or with change of atmospheric pressure or of humidity. In this category comes what has sometimes been called 'the healing breath' to be used when one needs a pick-me-up. This is the 1:4:2 technique described later in this chapter.

A third purpose of *prāṇāyāma* practice is to acquire the ability to set up and keep in motion during meditation a quieter kind of breathing than is usual during our active operations, as has already been explained. This breathing will supply the oxygen needed by the brain and body during the great quietness required for successful meditation. The reader will probably remember that in our chapter on 'Yoga and the Intellect' we have emphasized the necessity for 'attention without tension' in our description of how to meditate. Thus the breathing desirable during meditation is somewhat similar to that during sleep, in which the movement is slower and deeper and quieter than during ordinary wakeful activity. This condition should be practised, so that the yogi may know the feel of the mood of it, and be able to set it going at the beginning of his periods of meditation.

Posture is described before breathing in Patanjali's *Sūtras*. A mode of sitting suitable for meditation having been established, he says, the next consideration is regulation of the breathing. In this book I am putting breathing practices before postures, as it is intended for the West, where breathing exercises can be done by all regardless of particular postures.

Correct breathing is important. It is merely a commonplace to say that the average modern sedentarily-occupied person would do well for the sake of his or her future health and happiness to perform a few exercises to benefit the less used muscles. This applies particularly to the muscles of the chest, the abdomen, the neck, and the eyes. In the present chapter we are especially concerned with exercises in breathing – a matter which the teacher of elocution or of singing also finds necessary.

We may remember at the outset that the object of yoga exercises is never to produce athleticism, but only balance and healthy economy in the body. A discipline is needed for this. Some opponents of yoga have said that they prefer naturalness to discipline, overlooking the fact that people have become very unnatural, and that the so-called natural-ness is only habit in any case. There are some people who consider it natural to do many things which are nothing better than bad habits of action, thought, and emotion. Taste-enjoyments – to take an example – are often acquired. In the yogi the aim in external living is wise orderliness, in-telligence in all things, including breathing, and this in its turn is regarded as only a jumping-off place for the achieve-ment of a new, additional, spiritual wisdom to be arrived at through intuition (*pratibhā*). This sort of naturalness is seen in the treatment of breathing by Patanjali.

In the *Yoga Sūtras* very little is said about the details of breathing. It prescribes that posture or sitting should be steady and pleasurable, with a minimum of disturbance. We next see that Patanjali had the same attitude towards breathing. With regard to physical conditions he only wanted such as would conduce to successful meditation. His yoga is *rāja-yoga* – the term *rājā* (king) implying self-mastery, mind over body and will over mind.

Other schools there were and are which have one or other of two different ends in view – the good health of the body and the awakening of the body's latent powers. These are classed together as *hatha-yoga*. *Ha* and *tha* are taken usually to refer to the 'sun and moon breaths', though by a few there is the interpretation of it as 'the forceful yoga', from the word *hatha*, which means a stroke or blow (verb *han* to 'strike').

The classical works dealing mainly with breathing practices (*prāṇāyāma*) and postures (*āsanas*) are the *Hathayoga Pradīpikā* (*Light on the Hatha-yoga*), the *Gheranda Sanhitā* (*Gheranda's Compendium*), and the *Shiva Sanhitā* (*Shiva's Compendium*).

These works go into much detail as to various modes of breathing, which we will describe. But first let us study the main principles with Patanjali. In his teaching *prāṇāyāma* is given as a limb (*anga*), the fourth of the eight limbs of yoga.[1]

When Patanjali comes to describe the practice of *prāṇāyāma* he makes it clear that by the word *prāna* he means the ordinary breathing of the body, in which air is taken in and let out again alternately. There are three aphorisms (*sūtras*) dealing with the subject as follows:

Prāṇāyāma is the division or separation (*vichchheda*) of the movements of inbreathing and outbreathing. The condition (of the breath) as outgoing, incoming, and standing still, observed as to place, time, and number, becomes lengthy and fine. A fourth (condition arises) which casts aside the business of external and internal.[2]

Place refers to the movement of the air outside the body, measured from the nose. Time refers to the slowness or rapidity of it. Number refers to the relative lengths of time allowed for inbreathing (*pūraka*), holding the breath (*kumbhaka*), and outbreathing (*rechaka*). Fineness refers to the fact that the breathing should not be rough, forceful, or noisy, but should have a quiet, smooth, natural flow. The fourth condition, in which one is not thinking about inbreathing, holding the breath, or outbreathing, is suitable for meditation.

Regular breathing during meditation is not supposed, however, to *assist* the meditation. The object is to enable one to carry on the meditation without having to counteract the disturbances caused by irregular breathing. Indeed, some have found during deep thought a tendency of the breath to stop or pause with the lungs empty until a gasp and sometimes even a choke occurs. As a result of the good

1. *Yoga Sūtras*, ii, 29.   2. *ibid.*, ii, 49–51.

breathing habit, however, these troubles cease, and, as
Patanjali puts it, 'The covering of the light is diminished.'[1]
Or we could translate it as 'the obscuration of the clearness
is diminished'. Patanjali adds, 'and there is fitness of the
mind (*manas*) for concentration'.[2]

There is also another kind of importance of good breathing during meditation. It prevents the mind from injuring
the body. If the body is at all in a state of strain or tenseness,
which could be due to disordered breathing or inversely
could be a cause of disordered breathing, it will become
worn down by the meditation, whereas rightly it should be
rested and refreshed. It is for this reason that one often hears
the quotation, 'There is no *rāja* without *hatha*', the assumption being that everyone needs some correction in the
matters of sitting and breathing. The idea then is, as the
great Shankarāchārya said, that *hatha-yoga* is only intended
for those who need to be purged of impurities.[3] This is emphasized in the *Hathayoga Pradīpikā*, where it says that the
various practices of *hatha-yoga* have their ending when they
result in *rāja-yoga*.[4]

Patanjali gives no inkling as to his own views on this
point. Probably he considered that this may quite legiti-
mately differ in different persons, according to their con-
stitutions and past habits. The *hatha-yogis*, however, very
strongly recommend the practice of allowing a certain
period of time (e.g. two seconds) for inbreathing (*pūraka*),
four times that long for pausing with the breath inside
(*kumbhaka*) and twice the time of inbreathing for breathing
out (*rechaka*).

The words *pūraka*, *kumbhaka*, and *rechaka* mean respectively
'filling', 'pot-like', and 'expelling', as already explained. The
value of reciting these words and using their syllables for
the count of three, twelve, and six is that the student's mind
is kept on the ideas of inbreathing, holding, and outbreathing, whereas the counting of numbers or the reciting of
other meaningful words takes part of the attention away

1. *ibid.*, ii, 52.   2. *ibid.*, ii, 53.   3. *Aparokshānubhūti*, 144.
4. *Hathayoga Pradīpikā*, i, 67.

from what is being done. In further exercises other words or methods may be used, once the breathing rhythm is well established.

A student of yoga has only to practise this 1:4:2 method a little while to realize that though it may be an excellent practice for cleaning out the lungs and learning full breathing, it cannot be made the general habit of breathing to be adopted for meditation, during which one should, of course, forget all about breathing. In that undertaking, one should not think about breathing, any more than about digestive processes, or the beating of the heart. Breathing must be relegated to the region of bodily habits or the subconscious mind.

Breathing exercises are, however, desirable at other times for the sake of general health, because most people habitually breathe badly, just as they habitually walk badly and talk or enunciate badly. Bad breathing is undesirable in meditation even more than in daily life, because in the latter there are times of varied activity in which special efforts are occasionally made which cause deeper breathing and clean out the lungs, while there are no such correctives during meditation.

The breathing to be made habitual for meditation purposes should be a little slower than the breathing during activity of any kind. The student can test or check the number of complete breaths he takes in one minute. While doing so, he may observe whether he fills the lungs reasonably full, whether he breathes out fairly completely, and whether he breathes in again as soon as he has breathed out. Then, while practising to breathe a little slower than before, he may observe carefully that he mentally demarcates the three things just mentioned. The reduced amount of breathing due to slowness will be compensated by better breathing, and by the quietness of the body during the meditation. In this he must remember the overall rule in meditation – attention without tension.

The 1:4:2 breath has sometimes been called a healing breath. The beginner is recommended to do it only once or twice a day, and then only a few times. For most people ten times would be an ample maximum, to be reached gradually. In the beginning the unit of time can be conveniently measured by the recital of the word *pūraka* mentally once. Then, while holding the breath, comes the recital of *kumbhaka* four times, and next the recital of *rechaka* twice while exhaling. A certain amount of conscious effort will be needed to fill the lungs well in the period allowed. Then in the 'holding' of the breath with the count of four, one must not as it were cork the breath in at the throat, but simply be conscious of the chest muscles used in breathing, and let them be (tell them to be) inactive while there is the recitation of the *kumbhaka* four times at the same rate as with the *pūraka* while inhaling. In the third movement, an effort will again be needed to expel the air so quickly as to empty the lungs with the count of two *rechakas*. Then comes something to remember and attend to – the next *pūraka* must begin the very moment that the *rechaka* is finished, with no pause. When this whole process has been followed, say, three times, the student will probably 'feel nice', as the expression is. When all this is done with ease, he may, if he wishes, double the time, by reciting two *pūrakas*, eight *kumbhakas*, and four *rechakas*, and so on.

There is a question as to whether the reader of such a book as this who wishes to make some improvement in his life by means of yoga practice should do *prānāyāma* and other *hatha-yoga* exercises, and if so how much. This has to be answered by the enquirer himself. There are no rules in the matter, and, besides, making one's own decisions is a vital part of the advancement in yoga. I would say to one who desires to try, 'Do something – not too much – and one thing will lead to another.'

There is really a three-fold decision to be made at the outset – what proportion of time will be given to (1) *hatha-yoga*, (2) *rāja-yoga*, and (3) *ātma-yoga*. If the aspirant feels that his bodily condition is good enough for him to omit *hatha-yoga* altogether he may do so, and proceed with his *rāja-yoga* meditations. It is in such a case usually considered that his finding himself in that felicitous position is the result of his practices in former incarnations.

When deciding what *prānāyāma* to do, and how much of it, the student is *seriously warned* to proceed slowly and carefully and not to mix it with any emotional excitement, such as 'feeling on top of the world'. In this matter, the rule that enjoins one to do the work and not at the same time think about the results of it, is adamant. This warning is not new. The *Hathayoga Pradīpikā* says:

By proper practice of *prānāyāma*, etc., there comes the fading away of all diseases; by adherence to wrong practice there is the arising of all diseases – various diseases (including) hiccough, asthma, cough, pains in the head, ears, and eyes. Carefully one should exhale the air; carefully inhale it; carefully hold.[1]

In India the student often seeks a teacher (*guru*) whom he visits occasionally, and this is sometimes possible also in a few other places. Guidance thus obtained can be valuable, but here too there is danger. One should know a *guru* very well before blindly obeying any instructions he may give – know his character and motives especially, and if possible his effect on earlier students. It is true that the teacher will tell the student what to do and let him find out the benefits. He will not explain much beforehand, except in the *hathayoga*, in which the results are physically describable and have been known previously or seen in other persons, but care has to be taken not to be caught by teachers who are not conscientious, but are merely setting up in this field to get rich quick, or to feel important. And he must beware, as the sage Rāmakrishna said, of unripe *gurus*.

In most of the old books there is advice to seek a teacher. There was a very good practical reason for this in the old days – most people could not read, did not want to read, and saw no reason why they should read. To be able to read and write was, in fact, regarded as a social stigma in some places – the rich man did not do it, but employed servants, who were always at his beck and call, for that work.

1. *ibid.*, ii, 16, 17.

For most modern people the books now printed in large numbers are the *gurus*. Indeed, near the beginning of many standard classical works on yoga one finds the statement that an aspirant should seek a *guru*, but this is followed immediately by an account of what the *guru* will advise, and what he will teach. The *Gheranda Sanhitā* opens with an account of an aspirant's approaching Gheranda, and asking to be taught the *ghatastha-yoga*.

Ghatastha-yoga meant the yoga of the physical body, since *ghata* means a pot or vessel, and this body is the pot or vessel in which we keep our tools for living, such as the sense organs and the action organs. Incidentally, the student must take care not to think of the body as a vessel in which he is *confined*, since it is constantly asserted that a man can be free of it or free in it whenever he wills to be so, if he *really* desires to live by his own will and not yield to the lures of pleasure and pride which enslave him to the world.

As soon as asked, Gheranda replied in some generally instructive verses, and then proceeded to an extensive description of seven exercises pertaining to the requested yoga;

Good, good, O great-armed[1], this which thou hast asked. I will tell it to thee, my child. Attend to it with great care.

There is no trap like illusion, no greater strength than yoga, no greater friend than knowledge, no greater enemy than pride (or, the desire to be pleased with oneself).

Just as sciences may be learned by practice of the letters of the alphabet (in the beginning), so realization of the Truth (*tattwa*; the Thatness) is obtained by means of yoga.

According to (their) good and bad deeds the bodies (*ghatas*) of living beings are obtained. Action arises through the body. Thus rotates the body-mechanism.

Up and down goes the body-mechanism, just as from the power of the bulls (in the case of water being drawn from wells). Just like that, from the power of action (karma) the living beings rotate through births and deaths.

Like an unbaked (earthen) pot put into water, the body constantly is growing old. One arrives at excellence (lit. purity) of body, having baked it in the fire of yoga.

1. A compliment.

The seven accomplishments for the body are purity, firmness, solidity, steadiness, lightness, sensitiveness, and undefiledness.[1]

In the next two verses, Gheranda lists the seven accomplishments, of which *pranayama* is the fifth – that which gives rise to lightness.[2]

The reader may very rightly ask: Why all this preoccupation with the body, if the aim is to reach independence with reference to the body even while using it, and at last to reach ultimate living without it, in some other conditions which we may tentatively call spiritual?

The answer is that the body is to become the means to this freedom or independence. Suicide would be of no help. In Western parlance, the soul grows by doing the job of making bodily life a success, which is not done by negatively enjoying pleasures, but is rather like the work of an artist who is intent upon producing a perfect picture, but is really (without thinking of it – and probably it is best that he should not think of it) producing a perfect artist. Not that there will be no pleasures while performing this task – far from it, for with a body improved by yoga practice there will be the constant pleasure of health, felt as such, and in the use of the senses.

Some people say that there is a great deal of selfishness involved in this attention to one's own body, when the time could be spent in being helpful to others. The necessity for such helpfulness, however, arises mostly from the absence of such care on the part of the persons needing to be helped, and it would often do them much more good to see someone physically enjoying the benefits of right living. Besides, too many good people themselves become in due

---

1. *Gheranda Sanhita*, i, 3–9.
2. The other six are:
   (1) Six actions, leading to purity.
   (2) Posture (*asana*), leading to firmness.
   (3) Exercise (*mudra*), leading to solidity.
   (4) Sense-withdrawal (*pratyahara*), leading to steadiness.
   (6) Meditation (*dhyana*), leading to sensitiveness.
   (7) Contemplation (*samadhi*) leading to undefiledness.

course a burden to others because of neglect of themselves.

The recommendation of the *Bhagavad Gītā* that people should carry on their own respective social functions perfectly well represents the yogic attitude to our collective living, and at the same time indicates the road to that awakening of inner character and ability which will lift the future races of humanity. All human problems, both individual and social, have to be dealt with from the inside, always remembering that the pictures perish but the artist goes on.

This idea, that our works perish but we go on, and the improvement of the work involves the improvement of the worker, is one of the revolutionary ideas which the yoga philosophy brings to the West, which is so intent upon outward success or gain. Whenever there is trying there is the real success. The Western saying 'It is better to have loved and lost than never to have loved at all', could be paralleled with 'It is better to have tried and failed than never to have tried at all'. The reason for this is that there can be no failure in the yogic sense, as long as there is trying. Also to this must be added: the inward gain is carried forward to the future as greater ability, and so leads later on even to the comparatively despised outward success.

What, then, it is often asked, should be advised for beginners who have done no breathing exercises before? Probably some breathing connected with activity, on the principle that it is not good to do two new things at once.

One student was advised to go for half an hour's smart walk early morning, breathing in for eight paces and then out for eight paces. Testing this afterwards with the seconds hand of a clock he found that his count of eight usually occupied five seconds. He also found that he felt and was better in health than before. No doubt his entire breathing habit was improved.

While walking he was breathing deeply, quite instinctively, but suppose the same count had been followed while he was very quietly sitting or lying down, which he actually did later in the morning each day. He then soon found that he would need less 'filling' than when walking. Therefore his exercises while sitting came to consist of a slower intake of his normal amount of air, and not the filling of the lungs to capacity, as when walking briskly. In the two cases he was learning different lessons of breathing.

The result of such practice should be that after a while the student could switch from one to the other by a slight act of will, and the process of breathing then established would carry on in that manner without attention until changed by circumstances or by a change in the will or intention. It is to be remembered that the will is the 'carry-on' function of the mind, and can operate 'as set', so 'Now is the occasion for quiet breathing' or 'Now is the occasion for full breathing' would be obeyed until the order or command was changed.

Some such preliminary exercises are recommended for let us say two weeks or a month to all who are proposing to try some regular *hatha-yoga* breathing practices. Then the chest muscles will have been awakened from sluggishness to activity – a change in pleasurableness, fundamentally – and to responsiveness to the mind, though not yet, perhaps, to wise or intelligent rhythm. It is worth noting in this matter that the transition is ultimately to be from laziness to wisdom, which is intelligent orderliness, not to excited activity. This follows the triple training which the yoga system applies to almost every discipline – the triple course beginning in sluggishness (*tamas*), going on to activity, even restlessness (*rajas*), and ending in orderliness (*sattwa*).

The student may now wish to try some of the *hatha-yoga* special breathings and there is no reason why he should not do so in strict moderation, without any emotion, without any tension, and without ever drawing upon his adrenal reserves. If he disobeys these four rules he will have trouble. I know that some people follow 'courses' in which each exercise is preceded by a 'pep talk' and great expectations are engendered and excitement whipped up, and I know also that quite standard exercises done in those conditions have resulted in trouble.

Those who have at all understood the physiology of breathing will probably refrain from going to excess in any of the special yoga breathing exercises. It cannot be too strongly reiterated that there should *never* be any calling upon bodily reserves in these (or any other) exercises. When what is called 'forced breathing' results in tremors, dizziness, numbness, tingling, etc., it is time to stop, for the carbon dioxide has probably been reduced to half its normal – and similarly, holding the breath to the point of causing a warm flush in the skin or pounding of the heart is not advised. Bodily reserves are intended for emergencies and are definitely limited. If drawn upon to the limit they may be expected to be followed by a breakdown in whatever may be the weakest part of the bodily mechanism.

I recall a case which came to my notice of a man who was doing the breathing exercises prescribed by an advertising firm, and had suddenly been struck blind in the midst of enjoying one of them. On looking at his sheets of instructions I found some more or less well-known breathing exercises prescribed, but they were all preceded by an exciting emotional build-up calculated to induce the student to go to the limit in his effort. This evidently resulted in the exhaustion of his reserves and at that point a breakdown.

In the *Shiva Sanhitā*, a simple form of the alternate nostril breathing is given. I have translated it in somewhat abridged form as follows:

The wise man, having closed the right nostril with the thumb of the right hand, and having drawn air in through the left nostril, should hold his breath as long as he can, and then let it out through the right nostril slowly and gently. Next, having breathed in through the right nostril, he should retain the air as long as possible, and then breathe it out gently and very slowly through the left nostril. Let him thus practise regularly, with twenty retentions, at sunrise, midday, sunset, and midnight, every day, keeping a peaceful mind, and in three months the channels of the body will have become purified. This is the first of four stages of *prānāyāma* (regulation of breath), and the signs of it are that the body becomes healthy and likeable and emits a pleasant odour, and there will be good appetite and digestion, cheerfulness, a good figure, courage, enthusiasm, and strength.

There are, however, certain things which the *swāra-sādhaka* (breath-practiser) must avoid: foods which are acid, astringent, pungent, salty, mustardy, and bitter, and those fried in oil, and various activities of body and mind: bathing before sunrise, stealing, harmfulness, enmity, egotism, cunning, fasting, untruth, cruelty to animals, sexual attachments, fire, much conversation, and much eating. On the contrary, he should use and enjoy *ghi* (butter clarified by simmering), milk, sweet food, betel without lime, camphor, a good meditation-chamber with only a small entrance, contentment, willingness to learn, the doing of household duties with *vairāgya* (uncolouredness), singing of the names of Vishnu, hearing sweet music, firmness, patience, effort, purity, modesty, confidence, and helping the teacher. If there is hunger, a little milk and butter may be taken before practice, but there should be no practice for some time after meals. It is better to eat a small amount of food frequently (with at least three hours' intervals) than much at once. If the body perspires it should be well rubbed (with the hands). When the practice has become well established these rules need not be so strictly observed.[1]

Such are general rules suitable for the Indian climate and environment. In this exercise, when it directs that the air be retained 'as long as possible' it means 'as long as possible comfortably', that is, while still retaining the power to let the air out gently and slowly. One must not struggle, as it were, to prolong the retention. It is customary, while retaining and before releasing the breath to use the two middle fingers of the same hand to close the left nostril, and so on. Letting the air out gently means so that it will not flutter a bit of cotton held two or three inches from the nose. It is not desirable to do twenty retentions the first time, but perhaps five.

Modern teachers recommend the student to think of health, purity, goodness, etc., while breathing in. Some advise thinking of sending away all diseases, impurities, and vices, while breathing out, but others maintain that thoughts of anything bad should not be entertained, and in the course

1. Wood, Ernest, *Great Systems of Yoga*, pp. 89, 90.

of breathing out one should send out thoughts of health and good to all creatures, or to cases of special need. Be careful, it has been said, to keep a serene face.

As a second exercise, after the foregoing has been done at least once daily for about a month, the counting of 1:4:2 may be introduced into the same exercise, as described earlier in this chapter. First it should be done several times with both nostrils open, and then the method of alternate nostrils, using the thumb and fingers as before, may be taken up.

The counting may preferably be, as already explained, by the syllables of one recited '*pūraka*' for the inhalation, four recited '*kumbhakas*' for the retention, and two recited '*rechakas*' for the exhalation, which may perhaps be doubled or even further increased later on if desired. The reciting will be only mental, of course.

The student should be guided by his feeling of well-being (not of excitation) in deciding the number of rounds to do, and the number of seconds or units of time to use in the length of each movement. Statements appear now and then regarding yogis who continue such exercises for a long time, with very high counts. The voluntary suspension of breath has its limits, however. Entire voluntary inhibition is considered by scientific men to be impossible, and would amount to suicide by refusing to breathe, if it could be done. In this respect, breathing can be more voluntary than, say, digestion, but still within limits.

The general principle is that breathing is a habit, subject to change by practice which in turn produces a change of habit – and subject to voluntary suspension for short periods. It is considered that the average person can hold his breath for about three-quarters of a minute, and then the involuntary habitual condition reasserts itself despite his most determined efforts. The immediate cause of this, no doubt, is nerve impulses, not the muscules of the chest which as everyone knows, do not act when there is nerve injury such as occurs in some cases of poliomyelitis, even though they themselves are in perfect condition.

It is the impulses from the respiratory neurons located in the medulla-oblongata which give rise to the alternate activity and inactivity of the appropriate chest muscles. Those neurons are affected by various factors, including the relative chemical influence of oxygen and carbonic acid gas in the air in the lungs, the stimulation of the afferent nerves anywhere in the body, and also impulses from the upper brain (cerebral cortex) due to various emotions.

Our emotions thus play an important part in influencing the movements of the breathing process. It is part of the yoga psychology to say that *all* our ideas are accompanied by feelings and emotions, however slight.[1] These in turn normally affect our breathing as a result of their calling for some action – such as flight or fight in the case of fear – but one of the aims of yoga practice is to stop this effect while sitting in meditation and to be able to control it at other times. Thus, a yogi involved in an altercation which would usually give rise to indignation or anger can be perfectly calm. This often involves a momentary control of breathing which is perhaps not noticed.

Involuntary brief changes in one's habitual rate and volume of breathing are constantly taking place whenever one is awake and responsive to incoming impressions and to the flow of ones own thought and imagination with its attendant feelings. From both sides, then, the neural impulses of breathing are being influenced, and the background in both cases is a call to action. Let us be clear about this – the regular process of breathing is there to provide for the needs of metabolism, and has been very well established through the ages by dint of heredity and natural selection (the elimination of the unfit). It is very much disturbed by modern living, and sometimes a bad habit of breathing becomes established.

The yogi wants to (1) replace the bad habit by a proper and healthy one, and (2) keep off those afferent and emotional disturbances while he meditates and also, in the cases of the non-beneficial ones, at all times. For the last of these

1. *Yoga Sūtras*, i, 5.

purposes he practises *pratyāhāra* (control of the senses) and *samatwa* (equanimity of mind). Equanimity has been discussed in earlier chapters. Control of the senses will follow in our Chapter 7.

It is worth noting that in inbreathing the air is sucked into the lungs by the expansion of the thoracic cavity, and the consequent filling of the lungs from the atmospheric pressure outside the body through the channels of the nose (or mouth) and the windpipe (trachea). In outbreathing there is no such action, the chest muscles simply relax and fall back into their previous position. Even so the process does not continue to the extent of completely emptying the lungs; the emptying may be only, say, half effected when another impulse from the neurons in the respiratory centre sets the chest muscles going again into the act of contraction necessary for expanding the thoracic cavity. Incidentally, the diaphragm below the lungs, between the lungs and the viscera, is lowered by the pressure of the incoming air and returns to its original place by its own elasticity when the air is breathed out.

Therefore in the exercises in which it is desired to hold the air in the lungs for a while (called *kumbhaka* in the yoga terminology) or in which it is desired to prolong the period of expiration (*rechaka*), there is an inhibition or partial inhibition of the usual muscular release. In very fully filling the lungs there is a prolongation of the muscular contracting process which enlarges the cavity. In the extra emptying of the lungs there is the inhibition for a while of the recurring contraction of the muscles, so that the relaxation has fuller scope. In apparatus for artificial respiration, such as the 'iron lung', there is no pumping of air into the lungs, but only an alternation of increased and reduced air pressure on the outer walls of the chest.

In actual practice of *prānāyāma*, therefore, the student is recommended to be conscious of the muscles at the sides of the chest. If holding the breath in, he should be aware of keeping those muscles quiet, inhibiting their relaxation. The method of corking the air in at the throat, or clamping the trachea (windpipe) at the end of an inspiration, is not so desirable, as it can so easily result in a conflict or undesirable pressure when the chest muscles fall back and the 'cork' refuses outlet.

Incidentally, it is found in practice that when the lungs have been supplied for a little while with an extra amount of air (either by depth or rate of breathing) there is an automatic tendency to a compensatory suspension of inbreathing for a while. This is ascribed to an unusually great elimination of carbonic acid gas (carbon dioxide) and a reduction below the normal pressure of this gas in the blood. In experiments in 'forced breathing' in an atmosphere containing more than the usual amount of carbon dioxide the suspension effect is not found. When, on the other hand, the atmosphere is extra rich in oxygen, the experiment shows an increased suspension effect. As regards the increase of oxygenation of the arterial blood by such 'forced breathing', it has been found to be very little.

All this shows that excess breathing does not improve the oxygen supply in the blood (unless there has been some deficiency). This is also borne out by the fact that our outbreathed air normally contains a considerable amount of the oxygen breathed in, returned unchanged to the outer air. The amount of oxygen required by the blood varies, however. When there is great muscular activity, the amount of air taken into the lungs in one breath may be as much as four times as great as the normal, and the rate of the respiration twice the normal. Everyone has noticed, for example, how runners gasp and pant for breath, not because they do not breathe deeply and quickly, but because in such extreme efforts they still do not get enough oxygen.

The question naturally arises as to whether in meditation there is need for an increase of oxygen, as in physical exertion. On the principle of 'attention without tension' we assume that the need in proper meditation would be nothing like that in common thinking, in which there is (by sheer bad habit) a great deal of tension in various parts of the body. In proper meditation there is obviously need for less oxygen and this is no doubt the reason for the yoga instruction (empirically arrived at) that the breathing must 'become lengthy and fine'.[1]

One thing stands out clearly in the yoga systems of the *rāja-yogīs*, such as Patanjali – the principle of physical economy of energy. Thus it applies to breathing where the aim is to obtain *the right amount* of oxygen with the minimum of energy expenditure, so that the meditation can go on for a long time, if desired, without the tendency to sleepiness which would result from fatigue.

It should be taken into account that sleep becomes not needed when the expenditure of energy in wakefulness is reduced below the amount of expenditure of energy normal during sleep. There is always expenditure, whether a person is sleeping or awake. The calorie lists show that in normal persons the expenditure of energy during eight hours of sleep is about 600 calories. In the same period of rest it is about 750 calories. Suppose that in yoga one can be more relaxed than in ordinary sleep and reduce the above calorie expenditure below 600, then one may carry on without sleep. But in the case of the non-yogi there is not much real rest even when one is sitting thinking, as there is always some tension, and sometimes very much.

Therefore if the yogi can perform his 'attention without tension' well enough he can continue his meditation without sleep for a long time. If these figures are correct, we can see one of the reasons why after meditation the body can feel positively refreshed. We see, in fact, that it is possible to produce in meditation and in relaxation a condition *better* than normal sleep – more enjoyable and more refreshing.

This condition may also be one of the factors having a bearing on length of life. In general it has been observed that the slower-breathing animals are generally less excitable and live longer than the faster-breathing ones. For instance, a hen breathes about thirty times per minute, a duck about twenty, a dog about twenty-eight, a cat about twenty-four,

1. *Yoga Sūtras*, ii, 50.

a horse about sixteen, a monkey about thirty, a tortoise about three.

It should be remembered that meditation is the very opposite of going to sleep. In it the concentration alerts the attention to its maximum and this maximum is then carried forward into the greater mental scope of the meditation process. If it is not so carried forward on any occasion of practice, the student should drop the meditation and start again with a new act, or even a new object, of concentration. We have designated the two stages as 'grip' and 'grasp' in an earlier chapter.

It may be noted before leaving this subject that neither in connexion with breathing and relaxation, nor mentally and emotionally, is our object to 'get away from this world'. Material objects serve to assist our consciousness to achieve its current maximum quality by their stable character. This is the value of the 'world' to the growing mental power. A music composer, for example, will capture and dwell upon a passage which comes into his head by playing it upon his piano and writing it down. He can then reproduce it and modify it as he wishes. All our phenomenal experience has this value, and when the yogic theory of a subtle (and even formless) mind evolving or growing towards maturity through a series of lives or incarnations is accepted, there is seen the reason for such experience. In this lies the utility of our living under the restrictions of material conditions. They help the act of concentration which is at the beginning of every voluntary mental effort.

To return to our physical study of the breath – we have still to consider the effect of holding it in. While the inflow and outflow of air should be 'regular', still an occasional practice of inner suspension (*kumbhaka*) has a cleansing value. We can see how this works, especially with reference to the alveolar air in the lungs. The lungs may be considered in three parts – the wider channels (the bronchi), then the narrower passages (the bronchioles), and lastly the very fine, even hair-fine, clusters of branchlets (the alveoli). A standard intake of breath by the average person occupies approximately two seconds. If it is 'shallow' it does not satisfactorily aerate the alveoli. Now, shallowness is not a matter of time or length of the inhalation, but of lack of strength and decisive action of the chest muscles, so there is here an important point to be considered by shallow breathers, and to be acted upon by means of some decisive muscle-toning and habit-forming exercise.

We may indicate the use of the *kumbhaka* by means of the following sketch, which shows the great difference in the size of the bronchial tree, A, in full expiration, and B, in full inspiration. Deep breathing takes in about eight times as much air as quiet breathing.

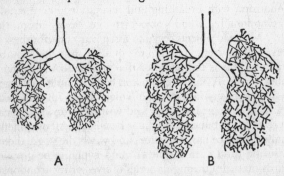

A   B

It must be understood that after full expiration the lungs are by no means empty of air. There will be let us say, in a given person (for cases differ) 150 cubic centimetres of air in the space from the nostrils to and including the bronchioles, which is termed 'dead space' because the air therein does not penetrate the relatively thick walls and produce any interchange of gases with the blood. After the expiration there will be, say, 200 c.c. of air remaining in the lungs. Now, in inhaling let us say that 500 c.c. of new air comes in. 150 c.c. of the mixture will still be in the 'dead space', and 350 c.c. will join the unexpired alveolar air, which is higher in carbon dioxide content and lower in oxygen content than the incoming air. A standard figure is that inhaled air contains 21 per cent oxygen and exhaled air about 12 per cent. The aeration of the blood is a big business, since the whole of the blood flows through the lungs in about 3 minutes, and amounts to one fifth of the entire weight of the body.

It is in the manner in which this incoming air arrives in the aureoles that one finds reason for the *kumbhaka* exercise. Experiments have been made which indicate that the diffusion or mixing of the inspired air (with its higher oxygen content and its lower carbon dioxide content) with the static air takes a little time. Further, the new air enters in the form of a cone in the centre of the duct, so that the old air still forms a layer on the inside walls of the tube until that diffusion takes place. This may be illustrated as follows[1]:

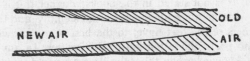

I take it that the *kumbhaka* allows of more perfect diffusion than would occur when the exhalation begins immediately at the cessation of the inhalation. The ratio of inbreathing (1 unit of time), holding (4 units), and outbreathing (2 units) which is generally followed and taught by the *hatha-yogīs* must, however, have been arrived at empirically, with a view to maximum benefit and operational economy, although it is thus seen to be scientifically sound.

Another benefit of this *prāṇāyāma* arises out of its insistence that when the outbreathing is complete (in twice the time of the inbreathing), there is to be no pause before the next inbreathing. This brings about a very conscious and even effortful inbreathing, which will help to counteract the tendency of some thinkers to pause at the end of an expiration before beginning the next inspiration, which in some persons takes place spontaneously until choking occurs. I remember a boy of fourteen years, whom I knew, with whom this not infrequently happened and was the cause of con-

1. After Yandell Henderson, in Best and Taylor's *Physiological Basis of Medical Practice*, p. 351.

siderable distress. He had a natural habit of falling into contemplation and it was in these circumstances that the choking occurred. The condition was cured in time by yoga breathing exercises.

In all the foregoing study we have not alluded to the possibility of stopping the breathing process after the *rechaka* or breathing out. There is a certain *hatha-yoga* practice, entitled *khecharī mudrā*, in which the tongue is thrust up into the nasal orifice at the top of the mouth and, the mouth being closed, taking in or letting out of air is completely prevented. The yogi then 'hibernates' for a long time, say forty days. Whether the yogi is sustained by the small amount of air taken in through the skin has not been ascertained, as far as I know. It is not stated in the books whether this is to be begun with the lungs filled or with them empty, and the old performers of the feat have, to the best of my knowledge, given no particular attention to this matter. In any case, modern knowledge has it that the lungs are never completely emptied of air.

Somewhat similar is the case of those persons who had ceased breathing but were still alive, including numerous cases of persons buried alive after being certified as dead. Coffins of persons buried alive which have been opened have disclosed evidences of the desperate struggles of such unfortunate people.

In describing the *khecharī mudrā* the *Hathayoga Pradīpikā* says nothing at all about the breathing, but explains that the tongue is turned up into the 'the hole in the skull', for which there is the preparatory task of lengthening the tongue.

It is possible to cut the attachment beneath the tongue, to assist this process. Details of the cutting are given: with a sharp knife the *fraenum lingum* is cut a hair's breadth at a time, and the cut is rubbed with powdered salt and turmeric. Thus says Swātmarāma, the author; but the commentator Brahmānanda remarks that as salt is prohibited for yogis they should use instead the burnt powder of certain kinds of wood. The tongue is then massaged and lengthened with the fingers, in a manner similar to that used in milking a cow. There is no suggestion of using any instrument for this, as in some books. The practice is repeated daily, but the cutting is mentioned as being necessary only once a week. The whole process requires six months. Some have stated that the tongue can be sufficiently lengthened for entering the inner hole without cutting at all.

There are always some men in India who do this and other abnormal things. There was a yogi Haridas who as a result of this practice could touch his forehead outside with his tongue. I have personally sat for a whole morning in friendly converse with a man who could stop the beating of his heart for a while and could also control the flowing of his blood, both of which he demonstrated to me.

Regarding the *khecharī mudrā* there is also an account in the *Gheranda Sanhitā*. I give a translation of this by Rai Bahadur Shrish Chandra Vasu of Allahabad:

Cut the lower tendon of the tongue and move the tongue constantly. Rub it with fresh butter, and draw it out (to lengthen it) with an iron instrument. By practising this regularly the tongue becomes long, and when it reaches the space between the eyebrows then the *khecharī* can be accomplished.

Then practise turning it upwards and backwards so as to touch the palate, till at length it reaches the holes of the nostrils opening into the mouth. Close the holes with the tongue (thus stopping inspiration), and fix the gaze on the space between the eyebrows. This is called *khecharī*.[1]

Shrish Babu has stated that it takes about three years to cut through the whole tendon, and that he saw his own *guru* doing it as follows: Every Monday he used to cut the tendon one-twelfth of an inch deep and sprinkle salt over it, so that the cut portion might not join together. Then, rubbing the tongue with butter, he used to pull it out with special iron instruments.

The term *khecharī*, by the way, means 'one who walks in the sky', or the ether. This relates, no doubt, to the idea

1. *Gheranda Sanhitā*, iii, 25-7.

that during trance a yogi may travel about 'in his subtle body'.

This travelling in the subtle body (*sūkshma sharīra*) is not to be confused with levitation, which means the floating of the ordinary physical body in the air. This is acquired, it is said, mainly by the practice of the 1:4:2 system of breathing, carried to great lengths, in some cases even to the extent of 36:144:72, counting these as seconds, or counting the 'time taken by a man to turn up his hand over his knee three times and snap his finger and thumb once' of some of the *gurus*. The method of the modern doctor who counts his seconds by 'thousand-and-one, thousand-and-two, etc.' might be more convenient.

Levitation, or the rising of the body from the ground and its suspension a few feet up in the air above the seat or couch, is a universally accepted fact in India. I remember one occasion when an old yogi was levitated in a recumbent posture about six feet above the ground in an open field, for about half an hour, while the visitors were permitted to pass sticks to and fro in the space between. Princess Pena Choki, second daughter of the Maharaja of Sikkim, related, regarding her uncle:

He was the most extraordinary man I have ever met. I remember that when I was a little girl he ... did what you would call exercises in levitation. I used to take him a little rice. He would be motionless in mid-air. Every day he rose a little higher. In the end he rose so high that I found it difficult to hand the rice up to him. I was a little girl, and had to stand on tiptoe ... There are certain things you don't forget.[1]

There are several other well-known breathing exercises which may be briefly mentioned to conclude this chapter. They are for occasional use and special purposes.

The Bellows (*bhastrikā*). The name given to this exercise is descriptive of its action. It is similar to one of the exercises occasionally employed by teachers of singing, and might almost be described as panting. A standard form of it is described as follows:

1. From Maraini, Fosco, *Secret Tibet*, London (Hutchinson), p. 52.

Just as the bellows of the blacksmiths alternately move in and out, so let one quickly move the air through both nostrils. Having done this twenty times one should perform a *kumbhaka*, and then expel the air by the previous method. The sensible person should perform this (whole) *bhastrikā-kumbhaka* three times.[1]

The *bhastrikā* is then praised as a means to good health and freedom from disease and bodily trouble.

The other exercises are variants on what have been described in this chapter. In some there is the drawing in of air through both nostrils, and expulsion through either right or left. In some there is the use of the tongue as a curved channel, while air is drawn in through the mouth. In some the breathing is done with sound, and in some there is forcible and even explosive expulsion of the breath. Often the exercises are done along with the use of *Om* and other *mantras*. Many variants have been added by numerous teachers during the centuries, and are being added even at the present time.

1. *Gheranda Sanhitā*, v, 75–7.

CHAPTER 6

THE POSTURES OF YOGA

THE term *āsana* or seat is used to connote a large variety of different postures which mostly involve bending and stretching the trunk of the body, and serve to keep it very supple. There is this vast difference between Indian and Western physical exercises – the latter are largely intended to develop muscular strength, the former not at all. In the yoga school, at any rate, the chief aim is to cultivate poise and balance which, whether in sitting, or in standing or in walking, will call for the minimum of muscular effort, and if possible no compensatory effort at all.

We may divide the postures into two groups: (1) those intended to be retained for a long time in meditation; (2) those intended for bodily fitness, most of which are meant to be retained for a very short time, in some cases only a few seconds.

In postures for meditation, 'head, neck, and back in a straight line' is the first requirement. Then 'the whole resting completely on the buttocks'. In this balanced position the legs may be folded in front in various ways. The straight line gives the feeling of 'sitting up' rather than 'sitting down'. The reader who will try these feelings will probably find that in passing from 'sitting up' to 'sitting down' there will be something of a slump.

The tyro is fairly sure to remark that the 'sitting up' will call for more energy than the 'sitting down'. That is quite an illusion. On the contrary, the body properly balanced uses no energy to keep upright, so that it becomes quite easy to sit still and forget it for, say, three hours, if desired, though meditation rarely requires such a length of time. And when the period is over and other duties call it will be found that the body is unwilling to move, being so happy in that highly relaxed condition that a definite act of will-power is needed to make it get up.

There are, however, some necessary conditions for success. One is that the neck must have the correct muscular development. Many people carry their heads crookedly all the time, not because of faulty connexions between the vertebrae (which an osteopath or a chiropractor can usually put right) but through sheer bad habit. In such a case the neck muscles need education by a series of exercises, a good set of which will be given at the end of this chapter.

A second requisite is that the shoulders should be habitually well held, which is a matter that can be put right while walking. They should not be strained back, of course, but on the other hand there should be no forward droop at all. One should feel the collar stud (old style) or the touch of the shirt or coat (new style) at the back of the neck, where it connects with the main part of the cervical column. Sedentary persons should test themselves occasionally at their desks.

After the neck and shoulders, the abdominal muscles need attention. They should be strong, and should every day receive some exercise – drawing them in and up and then lowering them again a number of times. This is a very rejuvenating exercise, and can be practised at odd times – while walking, in a car or train or bus, or on the toilet seat. If there is sleeplessness in bed at night, one can with benefit perform this exercise; being physical, it will conduce to sleep.

With this equipment one can sit greatly relaxed, either crosslegged or on a chair. It is necessary now that one should know the feel of relaxation. This is to be acquired first in a small part of the body, such as hand and fingers, then with the aid of that remembered feeling one can produce a relaxation all over, by a piecemeal process.

We will suppose (since this book is being published in England) that one is sitting on a chair. The chair must have a firm – not necessarily hard – seat, and must be of the correct height, so that the underside of the thighs can be quite horizontal while the feet are resting on the floor with a right angle at the knee. If the chair is too high, a stool may be put on the floor, women may wear high enough heels.

The feet may be fairly near together if when they are in that position the knees do not fall apart sideways during relaxation. If they do so, the feet are to be moved apart until the position is found in which they do not fall at all. People are structurally different in this respect. The legs may now be relaxed by an act of thought.

Next, one must see to the balance of the back by 'sitting tall', imagining a pull from above. It is usually desirable to stretch and shake the neck a bit and let it settle again to find the correct balance. See that the shoulders are all right, and now attend to the arms. This is done by letting them hang from the shoulders down the sides. Then, without altering the vertical position of the upper arms, bend the elbows and bring up the forearms until the hands rest on the thighs in their natural position according to the length of the arms. Now relax the arms entirely and let the thighs support all the weight of the forearms.

This being done, the student is ready for meditation.

Patanjali, our greatest authority, does not prescribe any special posture for meditation. He merely requires that it should be steady and pleasurable, and, we may add, healthy. Here are his aphorisms on the subject:

Sitting is to be steady and pleasurable. (This is done) by loosening of effort and thinking on the Endless.

Thence there is no disturbance from the pairs of opposites.[1]

Many teachers have their favourite postures, which they teach to their pupils – and many of the postures are very ancient – but Patanjali leaves the students to choose their own. The reference to the 'Endless' with a capital E, is to the symbol of the serpent of eternity – time is like a snake in that it glides along continuously without jerks. The god of life (Vishnu) is popularly depicted as reclining on this coiled-up serpent, which is sometimes pictured in the form of a serpent with its tail in its mouth especially to indicate the idea of continuity or endlessness, and therefore eternity, namely, the conception that time goes on as long as time

1. *Yoga Sūtras*, ii, 46–8.

exists,[1] though it can and will be withdrawn by the Deity when the aeon has gone on long enough.

When the student thinks of the Endless as he composes his body for meditation, he puts aside all thoughts of haste or outside pressure. Like the very god, he rides on time, and is not driven by it, so he can proceed without anxiety or the thought that he has to achieve something in a given time, or else fail. There is thus an emotional relaxation as well as a bodily one.

We will now give a description of the postures which are most favoured for meditation. The numerous authorities differ in opinion as to which is best, the well-known *Hatha-yoga Pradīpikā* approving of the *siddhāsana* above all others. The student may make his own choice if he sits on the ground, but if he sits on a chair he may follow the technique already described.

1. *Padmāsana* – the lotus seat

Sit with the legs out in front. Then bend the knees (with the help of the hands) so that the legs are folded, as it were, the left foot being on the right thigh and the right foot on the left thigh, both with the soles turned upwards. The hands are then rested on or near the knees. Some prefer the palms of the hands downwards and others turn them upwards with the tip of each index finger forming a circle with its thumb. The chin may be on the breast or held up. The gaze may be on the tip of the nose or straight in front (unfocused). The arms may be crossed behind the back with the hands holding the big toes. One variant is to place the palms together and rest them in the middle in front. Another (called *yogāsana* – the yoga posture) is that in which the hands are placed on the ground with the palms upwards.

2. *Siddhāsana* – the adept's seat.

In this case the knees are wider apart than in the lotus

1. An eternity is a period of existence of time. Before and after it there is no time.

seat, since one heel is touching the centre of the body in front (near the anus) and the other is just over its ankle. This causes the toes of the first foot to come between the calf and the thigh of the second leg. The hands on knees, the chin and the eyes may be placed as in *padmāsana*.

3. *Sukhāsana* – the pleasant seat

This is the easiest of all the *āsanas* and is intended for those who are too old or too stiff to be able to perform the other *āsanas*. In this case, after crossing the legs, raise the knees eight or nine inches above the ground. Then pass a scarf or folded cloth round the small of the back and round the legs below the knees and knot it in front so that the weight of the knees is supported by the cloth. The hands may then be put together palm to palm and rested on the cloth between the knees.

4. *Swastikāsana* – the auspicious seat

In this posture the left foot is placed between the calf and thigh of the right leg with the heel at the groin and the right foot is placed between the calf and thigh of the left leg. As an alternative, the left heel may be placed under the body end of the right thigh (at the groin), and the right heel over the body end of the left thigh. In this *āsana* care has to be taken not to lean to one side.

5. *Vīrāsana* – the hero posture

This is a very simple posture, having several variants. (1) One foot is placed on the other thigh.[1] (2) One foot is placed over the other thigh, and the other foot is placed *under* the other thigh.[2] (3) One foot is placed on the other thigh and the other foot is turned backwards (outward).[3] (4) The left foot is placed under the right thigh, the right foot being flat on the ground in front of the left ankle with the knee upright, with the hands locked in front of the right knee, or

1. According to *Trishikhi Brāhmana Upanishad*.
2. According to *Shāndilya Upanishad*.
3. According to *Gheranda Sanhitā*.

else with the left hand on the left knee, and the right fore-arm balanced on the right knee.[1]

6. *Gomukhāsana* – the cow-face seat

In this the ankles are crossed, the sole of the right foot is placed under the left buttock, and the sole of the left foot under the right buttock. Thus one is sitting on the heels, the feet being turned with the soles upwards. Indra Devi recommends that the fingers be hooked together in the middle of the back, one arm going over its shoulder and the other coming up behind with the elbow near the waist.

7. *Vajrāsana* – the adamantine pose

This term is applied by some to the *siddhāsana*. Others say that the right heel should be placed above the penis and the left on top of that. Others again apply the term to a posture which is like the prayer position of the Moslems, and also like the sitting pose often adopted by the Japanese. The two legs, with the knees fairly near together, have their lower parts bent back so that one sits on the heels, which are on each side of the anus. In this kneeling position the knees and insteps are on the ground, forming straight lines from the knees to the toes. This is a strain on the knees and ankle-joints which is overcome by practice and massage.

The foregoing postures have been put in one group to-gether because they are of the kind that can be continued for a considerable time, and therefore can be used in medi-tation. There is, of course, no special value for meditation in any posture. For this purpose only what is healthy, pleasant, easy, and economical of energy is desired. Different postures suit different people – those who are thin and loose-jointed, for example, can assume the lotus seat very easily.

The student who wishes to use one of these postures should try them out, select the one which suits him best,

1. A traditional pose for the warrior, often advocated for sitting at attention. It is considered to be a posture of readiness to spring into action, if that should be necessary.

and keep to that. There should be no thought that sitting on a chair is in any way inferior or discreditable. That would be mere superstition. Even lying down would be quite in order, but for the tendency – through mental and feeling habit – to sleepiness. The only disadvantage of the chair is that you have the trouble of owning it and you cannot take it about with you.

Some teachers and pupils are particular about the material to be used when sitting on the ground. There are often definite prescriptions in the authoritative books, though Patanjali gives none. On this subject the *Bhagavad Gītā* has the following verses:

Having settled in a clean place on a firm seat of his own, not too high and not too low, which has some *kusha* grass, a furry skin, and a cloth upon it – there, having made the *manas* (mind) one-pointed, with the senses and thoughts and actions controlled, having sat on the seat, he should practise yoga (meditation) for the purification of himself.

Holding body, head, and the back part of the neck properly (*samam*), unmoving, (and) steady, and having (next) looked in front of his nose without seeing in any direction, being himself quieted, with fears all gone, steady in the observance of Brahma-conduct, having poised the *manas* with me as (its) thought, let him sit, united, with me as (his) Beyond (*para*).

The yogi, with *manas* controlled, always meditating thus on the *ātmā*, arrives at my state, the nirvānic ultimate, which is peace.

But yoga is not for the excessive eater, and not for one who avoids food too intently, and not for one addicted to excessive sleep, also not to (excessive) wakefulness. Yoga becomes the destroyer of pain for one whose food and recreations are appropriate, whose efforts in action are appropriate, whose sleeping and waking are appropriate.

When the controlled mind (*chitta*) stays only on the *ātmā*, without longings for all objects of desire – then one is called united (*yukta*).[1]

1. *Bhagavad Gītā*, vi, 11–18. It should be mentioned with reference to the last of these verses that the *Gītā* is here prescribing for an advanced stage of the pupil. This is shown by the mention of the *Ātmā*, the supreme or inmost Self in every man. My reason for this statement is that the *Bhagavad Gītā* clearly teaches three definite grades in order. It begins

The use of a skin, a cloth, or the sweet-smelling and insect-repellant dried grass, the kind called *kusha* or *darbha*, is mentioned in various other writings, sometimes together and sometimes separately. It is not to be assumed that these are necessary to meditation; they are merely commonsense conveniences. A soft yet firm seat is desirable. In the natural, simple life people would normally sit on grass or earth, not on hard rocks or boards. The natural cushioning flesh on the human buttocks indicates the need for some softness, but does not sufficiently provide against hard material. It is a defect of old-style wooden chairs that they are too hard, and of the stuffed ones that they lack firmness, so probably when a chair is used the best is a wooden one, covered with a folded cloth. These remarks are not, however, to be applied in the matter of recumbent relaxation, which will be discussed under the heading of *shavāsana*, the corpse-posture, further on in this chapter.

It is important that, when the student works at accustoming himself to any of the postures – whether the foregoing seats or the still to be described gymnastic postures – he should never *force or strain* at all, but proceed gently and gradually. Little by little over a period of days or weeks of regular and brief trials he may come to the point where a posture is easy and natural. Never should outside help in the way of pressure by another person be allowed – the danger of strained tendons and torn ligaments is too great; one remembers the case of a man whose ankle was broken in an attempt to acquire too suddenly the position named 'the bow'.

the *Sānkhya Yoga* at Verse ii, 11, adds the *Buddhi Yoga* at Verse ii, 39, and after expounding that at length as right conduct and understanding of life in this world, definitely introduces the course of *Ātmā Yoga* in Discourse iv, with but slight mention of it before that (as in iii, 17–18) in reference to what is behind the *Buddhi-yoga* which is then being taught. The pupil's grief at the sorrows, indeed horrors, which he was then facing in this world of action had to be removed by (1) first, the *sānkya* knowledge of the relation between body and spirit as such (2) secondly, the *buddhic* knowledge of the value of life in this world, and (3) thirdly, the realization of the presence and meaning of *Ātmā*, the supreme Self.

The books list eighty-four postures (*āsanas*) altogether, but many of them are rarely used, some perhaps never. There are about a dozen of the gymnastic ones which are frequently used and which, in fact, would more than cover the ground required for health and functioning (in contrast with the partial atrophy so common in modern life) of all parts of the body. Most yogis, indeed, find it necessary to practise regularly only four or five.

First, we will present three *āsanas* requiring a head-down position, which are not uncommon in modern gymnasia:

1. *Shīrshāsana* – the head pose

This is what is commonly called standing on one's head, or the headstand, though, in fact, it is mainly a pose on the forearms along with the head, the arms taking part of the weight. There would, of course, be no gain in subjecting the crown of the head to undue pressure. The best procedure is to interlock the fingers of the two hands, and cup the back part of the top of the head between the hands, and use a folded cloth or pad.

Kneel down, lean forward, put the head and forearms on the ground, and gradually raise the body and legs which are at first bent, into the vertical upside-down position, with or without the aid of another person or a wall. The beginner may find it helpful to do this in a corner where two walls meet. Five minutes of this stand is usually recommended, twice a day. In many places some *hatha-yogīs* may be seen to do it for hours together, though that is quite unnecessary for any reasons of health.

Associated with this *āsana* there is another, named *ūrdhwa-padmāsana*, the upside-down lotus posture. In this, one stands on the head and forearms exactly as in the head pose, but folds the legs as in the lotus pose instead of keeping them straight up.[1]

1. We have not attempted to list the particular benefits to health which are assumed to be derived from these two *āsanas*, which would probably involve some encroachment on the domain of the medical profession, and would indeed if conscientiously carried out require a

2. *Sarvāngāsana* – the pose of all the limbs

This is done by lying flat on the back, then raising the legs and the back until one is standing on the shoulders. The help of the hands is needed, as the hands guide and support the raising body, and help to sustain the position by holding the body above the waist while the elbows and upper arms on the ground take a part of the weight. The chin is pressed against the chest and the legs are kept vertical. At first this pose can be kept for only about half a minute, but later on even up to four or five minutes. This, or something very similar – for in nearly all these practices different teachers have their variants – will be found again under the title *Viparītakaranī* among the *mudrās* in our next chapter.

3. *Halāsana* – the plough pose

Proceed as if about to do the *sarvāngāsana*, but let the legs continue over the head until the toes touch the ground. Then the arms will lie straight along the ground. The knees and legs should be kept straight. This pose also can be held from about half a minute up to four or five minutes. This exercise is by some carried further by bending the knees so as to bring them down to the ground on each side of the head, the hands now holding the calves.

Starting once more with the lying position we list a group of recumbent postures, most of which stretch the spine.

1. *Shavāsana* – the corpse posture

This is simply assuming the posture of a lifeless body, lying on the back with the arms along the sides. The real purpose of this exercise is to relax the entire body. It is usual to begin with the toes and legs, then relax the hands and arms, then the trunk, the neck, the face, paying attention to

great study of the work of the blood-pumping mechanism of the body, and many other things. Similarly, we will refrain from such comments in describing the subsequent *āsanas*, leaving it to the reader's common sense to recognize some of the benefits, and to his pragmatic conclusions when they are practised.

the chin, cheeks, and temples, and finally the scalp. This exercise is best done on a definitely firm ground, so that one has to go as limp as possible so as to have maximum contact with the floor, thereby reducing the pressure of the weight on the hard points where the bones are nearest to the surface. At the same time one should relax the emotions and thoughts, in order to get the best effect. Some teachers prescribe a little time to be given to this exercise after every course of yoga gymnastics. The refreshment derived from it is very great. These three relaxations – of body, emotions, and thought – should be done before going to sleep. The disadvantage of a soft bed is that on it a person may go to sleep without relaxing. On a hard bed relaxation is compulsory.

Relaxation plays a great part in yoga technique. In the *shavāsana* one can perhaps learn it as completely as possible. But the general idea is that when one part of the body is being used, the other parts should be relaxed as much as may be practicable. One form of relaxation is often neglected, that of the face, which should certainly be performed along with general relaxation before going to sleep. It can best be learnt while standing up. Lean the upper part of the body a little forward with the hands on the slightly bent knees. Then loll the head forward, relaxing all the muscles of the face and shaking it with little jerks (not too much) so as to feel the effects in the jaw, nose, cheeks, temples, etc.

2. *Pashchimottanāsana* – the drawing-back posture

Lie down with the legs stretched straight out together, without bending the knees. Then sit up without moving the legs, and continue the movement forward to take hold of the toes or to touch the insteps. This should be done without any jerking, and the head should continue to bend forward and downward until the forehead touches the knees, or the face is between the knees. This position should be held for only a few seconds at first, but later on may extend to minutes.

A half-way house to success in performing this posture is to do it first with one leg only, taking each in turn.

It will be of help to prepare for this important posture if one first does the 'Free-from-wind' exercise. This is done while lying down. One knee is then bent and brought up over the abdomen, while both hands clasp the leg below the knee and press it gently but firmly against the body several times. That leg is then released to the previous stretched-out position and the other is similarly treated.

3. *Matsyāsana* – the fish posture

This is a lying-down posture which is arrived at from the sitting position, preferably with the legs folded in the lotus-seat or similar manner. In this lying down, however, the middle of the back is not to touch the ground – only the posteriors and the top of the head should do that, with the back remaining in the form of an arch. The elbows may be used to enable one to acquire the position, and then the arms should no longer support the position but should be brought forward with the hands grasping the feet, or laid palms upward over them. The position may be held for, say, half a minute in the beginning and up to two or three minutes later on.

4. A posture much approved by Indra Devi of Hollywood is called by her the 'pelvic posture'. In this one sits in the kneeling position, but not with the heels under the body as described in one form of the *vajrāsana*, but with the feet wider apart so that they lie on each side, with the buttocks on the floor, and the arms down the sides with the palms resting on the ground. This is itself a posture, but is also carried further when one leans backward, with the help of the elbows, and lies with the back straight, and the arms either bent with the hands behind the neck, or stretched out.[1]

We will now give a group of *āsanas* which begin with lying down face downwards:

1. See, Devi, Indra, *Forever Young, Forever Healthy*, p. 156.

1. *Bhujungāsana* – the cobra posture

First, lying face downwards, one places the hands on the ground near the shoulders and, bending the elbows, pushes up or erects as much as possible the upper part of the body, above the navel, which should continue to touch the ground. The head is thrown back, stretching the neck. The position is retained generally from half a minute to a minute.

2. *Shalabhāsana* – the locust posture

In this one lies face downwards. First, with the chin on the ground and the arms extended alongside the body, one raises one leg up as much as possible without bending the knee, then lowers it and raises the other, then lowers that and raises both. In this position one then raises also the head and shoulders as much as possible. Retain the position for half a minute to a minute.

3. *Dhanurāsana* – the bow posture

Lie face downwards. Keeping the legs close together, bend the knees so that the feet rise up. Raising the shoulders, reach the arms backwards so as to catch hold of the ankles and pull them up away from the ground. The body will then be balanced on the abdomen. This position can usually be retained for only a quarter of a minute, but even so a few rocking motions may be made.

4. *Mayūrāsana* – the peacock posture

From lying down, take a kneeling position, bending forward, with the forearms near together, palms on the ground, the little fingers being beside each other, the fingers pointed towards the feet, and the elbows fitted close to the sides of the body. Keeping the legs stiff and straight and the head up, balance the body on the elbows, parallel with the ground. The position may be retained from a few seconds up to about two minutes. The position resembles the 'plant balance' of Western gymnastics.

5. *Kukkutāsana* – the cock posture

Although the cock posture is not a full-length one, I have

placed it next to the peacock posture because in these two *āsanas* the whole body is off the ground. The legs being in the *padmāsana* position, the hands are pushed down between the thighs and the knees, so as to raise the whole body, resting on the elbows, above the ground.

6. *Utkatāsana* – the raised or eager posture

In this the body is off the ground to the extent of being balanced on the balls of the feet and toes only. The heels are raised from the ground, and one sits on the heels.

There are some good postures for twisting the spine, of which the best known is:

Matsyendrāsana – the posture of Matsyendra[1]

The left heel is to be placed near the anus. The right foot is then brought over the left leg near the knee, with the right knee raised and the foot on the ground. Next, the hollow of the left armpit is to be fitted on over the right knee. The right foot is now to be held by the left hand. Now twist the spine, turning the body well to the right, the face being in line with the right shoulder. The right arm should go round to the back, with the hand holding the left thigh. Repeat the exercise on the other side. Repeat the whole two or three times.

The *matsyendrāsana* is very valuable as a spine-twisting exercise. For those who do not wish to sit on the ground, the following may be substituted: Stand with the back to an object ten or twelve feet away. Bend round slowly to the left so as to look straight at the object, at the same time moving the left leg forward and to the right. Move slowly back and reverse the process. Repeat several times. Simple exercises of leaning from side to side and also rotating the body from the waist are a good supplement to this. These may be done sometimes wearing a tight belt so as to emphasize the consciousness of the muscles.

1. Matsyendra was the name of the man who designed this posture or made it famous.

We will conclude with a few miscellaneous well-known postures:

1. *Muktāsana* – the liberated pose

This is simply sitting with the right and left heels touching – some say just touching and some say crossed.

2. *Bhadrāsana* – the prosperity pose

The heels are crosswise under the testes; the knees bound together by the hands, or the hands are crossed behind the back, holding the toes.

3. *Sinhāsana* – the lion pose

Sit on the crossed heels, with the hands on the knees, fingers stiff and stretched apart. The mouth is to be open, and the tongue stretched out towards the chin. The eyes also are wide open. This posture is extolled as good for sore throat.

4. There is a bow-string posture in which one sits with both legs extended, bends forward, and takes hold of the toes. Then, one arm being still extended, the other draws the foot towards the ear.[1]

5. The following rocking exercise is highly recommended by Indra Devi, especially before retiring to sleep. Sit with knees up and hands clasped under the knees. Lean forward, then roll back and return, several times.

6. *Vrikshāsana* – the tree pose

Stand on one leg. Lift the other leg forward and place the foot at the top of the other thigh.

For those who feel the need of more neck exercise, which is a most important matter among sedentary people – 'You are as young as your neck' – there are the practices of (1) moving the head from side to side with just a tiny little jerk at each extreme; (2) moving the head forward and backward without raising or lowering the chin at all; (3) leaning

1. *Hatha-yoga Pradīpikā*, i, 25.

the head over, first on one side then on the other; (4) lolling the head right forward with the chin on the chest, and backward with the mouth wide open and loose; (5) hanging the head forward loosely with the body leaning, then rotating the body so that the head rolls all round simply by force of gravity, first one way round and then the other way; and finally (6) stretching the neck upwards by a reaching movement of its own, with various little side movements to loosen it. The last is useful whenever settling into one of the postures for meditation. It straightens the neck and also the back.

CHAPTER 7

SENSE-CONTROL, PURIFICATIONS,
AND OTHER SUCH PRACTICES

As stated before, one of the first discoveries made by Western man on coming into contact with educated yogis and yoga literature was that here is a group of people who are not satisfied with themselves, but want to improve themselves – their bodies, their emotions, their mentality, their ethics and morality, and their spark of spirituality. Western man in general is apt to think that if he could improve his circumstances – increase his comforts, conveniences, and enjoyments and ensure his material safety and security – it would be enough and all would be well.

The Indian philosophers of long ago assessed the situation quite scientifically. That is why they were called *Sānkhyas*, which means people who enumerate and classify. The first item in their observations was that mankind is troubled and endangered by three kinds of things, classed as the material world, other living beings, and themselves – with, it may be added, the last as the worst.

Even the comparatively later Vedāntists, who had figured out what superior good awaits men, concluded that it was not enough for man to war and work upon his environment. In all respects he has to purify and develop *himself*. We are well aware that if the average man were suddenly transported from his condition of struggle into the lap of luxury and security (without any sort of restraint) he would soon begin to wreck himself. So far from gaining the heights of human enjoyment he would fall for many temptations.

Some time ago the American Bankers' Association studied the life experience of a hundred 'average men', who were all strong and vigorous, with good mental and physical capacity when at the age of twenty-five. Ten years later there were only ninety-five, of whom ten were wealthy and eighty-five not. Ten years still later only three wealthy ones were left, but there were still eighty-four of the others! Puzzle: find the men who are healthy, wealthy, and wise!

The young Vedāntist wants to prepare himself for an increase of the spark of spiritual understanding. At once he finds himself confronted by a programme of self-improvement set out in definite terms:

(1) Control of mind.

(2) Control of body.

(3) Renunciation of superstition and dependence – the idea that his advance can be helped or impeded by others – and therefore the cessation of resentment and antagonism.

(4) Acceptance of the idea that he must endure what comes and make the most of it without complaining, even to himself.

(5) The acquisition of confidence in the laws of life under which he finds himself, and also in himself.

(6) Cultivation of steadiness in the pursuit of these goals.[1]

It is prescribed that the six attainments must be preceded by the awkening of discrimination (*viveka*) and the use of uncolouredness (*vairāgya*), and followed by a great desire for freedom.

It is considered that these are the qualities of character needed by men in order to make their entire lives – even down to their material lives – lives of the spirit which is at the heart of man, the spirit whose flowering will be his fulfilment. These Vedāntists believe that the individual man can do it, and begin the work here and now.

It is only when these four qualifications (counting the six accomplishments as one) are to a reasonable extent acquired that the pupil of Vedānta is regarded as fit or competent (*adhikārī*) to proceed with the real knowledge-yoga (*jnāna-yoga*) of Vedānta. The procedure is then three-fold. First there is listening (*shravana*) to the teachings – which includes reading, of course. Next comes thinking about

1. From the *Viveka Chūdāmani*, by Shankarāchārya, verses 22–6, and subsequent explanations. The whole work contains 580 verses. Also listed in *Atmanātma Viveka* and other works by the same famous philosopher.

them (*manana*). Thirdly comes meditation (*nididhyāsana*) upon them, which includes the triple process of concentration, meditation, and contemplation given in the yoga system.

In general, in yogic circles much meditation is recommended. In this connexion it is a good plan when preparing to read on a particular topic to pause and think of all that one knows about it before actually starting to read, and again to pause before putting the book away and consider what new information or idea or experience has been gained, and how it fits in with what one knew before. This method is very beneficial for awakening the mind into a proper state of inquiry at the beginning, and leaving it in a proper state of coordination at the end. If this method of reading calls for will-power, that also is good, for thus the will also gets its exercise and awakening.

The yogis have their bodily exercises and sittings (*āsanas*), breathings (*prānāyāmas*), and control of the sense (*pratyāhara*). The *hatha-yogīs* have also a variety of purifications, exercises (*mudrās*), and controls (*bandhas*). Control of the senses, and these purifications, etc., may well be grouped together to form our present chapter.

Clearly the persons having the yogi temperament would say, if asked, 'We are not satisfied with ourselves. Indeed we are much more dissatisfied with ourselves than with the world. We feel that we need much more to get away from the defects of ourselves than from our environment. The thoughtless think that the troubles of the world are to be avoided and escaped from as much as possible, but we say it is ourselves we must avoid and escape from. We know that we have three sources of trouble in life – from Nature, from other men, and from ourselves. We emphasize the last of these three, which is the most ignored by people in general.'

As soon as a person of any religion catches a glimpse of the Beyond or the Divine – even if only represented in high ideals – he begins to long for more of it, to think of it, to imagine it, and to represent it by the outward reminder of ritual words and actions. He even goes to the length of hoping and imagining that words and ritual actions will help him to have more of this Beyond or Divine. But it is only when he realizes that it is not the outside world, or other people, but himself who is the source of his trouble, that he begins to become a real yogi.

When he has that realization and looks at himself – at his physical habits and ways of living, his thoughts about others and about himself, things which are revealed to him when he pays proper attention to what he is doing (just analogous to what a man does when in walking he feels the foot as well as the ground, and the feeling of the ground makes him feel the foot better) – he is shocked and disgusted at what he finds in himself every now and then.

Therefore it is that universally or in all religions the second natural step, following upon the perceiving of the existence of the divine (named *viveka* – discrimination – among the Hindus, and *manodwāravajjana* – the opening of the doors of the mind – among the Buddhists) is purification. The contrast is so terrible that this is the natural consequence. And then – to run ahead a little – the third stage, intuition and illumination, becomes possible, and indeed natural. But now in this chapter we are concerned with purification. And since 'trouble from ourselves' arises from both body and mind, both these things are to be dealt with.

The neatest statement about the purifications practised by the *hatha-yogīs* has been made in the *Gheranda Sanhitā*, where it says:

Purification (*shodana*) is by means of six kinds of action:
By means of posture (*āsana*) strength (*dridhatā*) comes about;
By means of exercise (*mudrā*), steadiness (*sthiratā*);
By means of withholding the senses (*pratyāhāra*), bodily calmness (*dhīratā*);
By ordering the breath (*prānāyāma*), lightness (*lāghava*);
By meditation (*dhyāna*), vision of oneself (*pratyaksham ātmanah*);
By contemplation (*samādhi*), unstainedness (*nirlipta*), and even freedom (*mukti*);
Undoubtedly (*na sanshayah*).[1]

1. *Gheranda Sanhitā*, i, 10, 11.

The six kinds of purifying action are: (1) general cleansing, (2) washing the intestines (*vasti*), (3) cleaning the nostrils (*neti*), (4) loosening the abdominal contents (*lauliki*), (5) clearing the vision (*trātaka*), and (6) clearing the skull (*kapālabhāti*).

Again, the first of these, the cleansing, is divided into four kinds, which are: (1) internal washing, (2) cleaning the teeth, (3) cleaning the throat cavity, and (4) purifying the rectum.

Of these again the first is divided into four groups: cleansing (*a*) by air, (*b*) by water, (*c*) by fire, and (*d*) by exterioration. The methods are as follows:

(*a*) Cleansing by air. Giving the mouth the form of a crow's beak, little by little suck air in, swallowing it, until the stomach is full. Then slowly expel it through the rectum.

(*b*) Cleansing by water. Leaning the head back, fill the mouth completely with water. Then swallow it slowly. Move it into the stomach and from there send it out below.

(*c*) Cleansing by fire. Cause the knot of the navel to press back against the spine a hundred times. It is considered that the region behind the navel is a place of fire or heat – food is 'cooked' somewhere behind there – and the pressing so many times no doubt increases the heat; hence the idea that this is a cleansing by fire.

(*d*) Cleansing by exterioration. Having performed the crow-bill act, fill the stomach with air, hold it there for a half of three hours, and then press it down into the middle path, the intestines. Then, standing in water as high as the navel, get out the intestines with the two hands and wash the tube until the dirt is removed, and when the tube is clean put them back into the internal cavity.[1]

The second of the four kinds of cleansing, which is cleaning the teeth, is more extensive than the term 'cleaning the teeth' would indicate, for it has five subdivisions, dealing with (*a*) the teeth and gums, (*b*) the tongue, to its root, (*c*) the gullet, (*d*) the pair of ears, and (*e*) the passage in the skull. These are:

(*a*) Cleansing the teeth. Rub the roots of the teeth (i.e.

1. *ibid.*, i, 17–24.

the gums) with the essence (i.e. juice or sap) of the acacia catechu (*khadira*) plant, likewise clean earth, until all impurities are removed. This should be done every morning by those who are versed in yoga, for the preservation of the teeth.

How contrary this and other recommendations which follow are to the self-injury, so highly publicized in the West, inflicted upon their bodies by some fanatics in India – very few compared with the vast numbers of the people in all occupations of life who do some of the standard yoga practices daily for the benefit of body and mind.[1]

(*b*) and (*c*) Cleansing the tongue and the gullet. With three fingers – fore, middle, and ring – operating together and inserted into the middle of the throat (i.e. gullet), slowly rub the base of the tongue and then wash out the phlegm impurity. After next cleaning the tongue with fresh butter, several times milk it (as it were), very gently pulling it with a metal instrument holding the tip.[2]

(*d*) Cleansing the ears. The instruction here is very brief. It says, 'With the first and ring fingers clean the two holes of the ears', and then mentions that when this is done regularly the internal sound will become clear. Quite often this is taken to mean that what are called the mystic internal sounds will be heard, but this is not justified, since the proper source of such sounds is elsewhere described as meditation in the heart centre.

(*e*) Cleansing the hole in the skull. Here it is the outside of the skull that is intended, for it says, 'With the thumb of the right hand rub (or massage) the hole of the forehead.' This hole is the depression between the forehead and the nose. It is quite usual for mothers to give this massage to their young children, and the practice is considered a help

1. It is to be remembered that in India lunatics have always been left at large, as long as they were not dangerous to others, and that in the West, as in the East, there have always been more religiously mad aberrations than any other kind.

2. This treatment of the tongue is the only example I can recall of the mention of an instrument or tool in the entire literature of yoga exercises.

in keeping the nasal cavities clear. The method is also considered to be helpful in the development of clairvoyance or interior sight. It is added that it should be done every day on awakening, after meals and at the end of the day.[1]

The third of the four kinds of cleansing is termed the 'heart-cleaning'. The term heart is, however, used in a very general way, for the interior of the chest, including the base of the throat. This group of cleansing practices is described as three-fold (a) by a stick, (b) by ejecting (vamana), and (c) by a cloth. The second is sometimes described as vomiting, but is not so, and might be more accurately described as gargling.

(a) *Cleansing by a stick.* With a stalk of plantain (*rambhā*), or of yellow sandal (or turmeric), or of cane (or reed), slowly moved down into the middle of the 'heart' and then slowly withdrawn, phlegm, bile, and other impurities are cleared out through the upper passage, that is, by the mouth.

(b) *Cleansing by gargling.* After meals, drink water deep into the throat; then, after looking upwards for a short time, expel that water (through the mouth). There is no mention of shaking the water, or of bubbling air through it from the lungs, as is common in European or American gargling, but in practice it is often done with quite a good deal of vehemence and noise.

(c) *Cleansing by a cloth.* Slowly swallow a fine cloth of a width of four fingers (about three inches), and then draw it out again. This is credited with being a help in trouble with phlegm or bile, and in various skin diseases.[2]

The fourth, and last, of the internal cleansings, the purification of the rectum (*mūla-shodhana*) is described as to be done with a stalk of the turmeric (or yellow sandal), or with the middle finger, made wet with plenty of water a number of times. This is declared to be a help against constipation and other digestive troubles.[3]

The group of *vasti* or *basti* (intestinal) procedures contains two kinds, wet and dry. The wet method compares

1. *Gheranda Sanhitā*, i, 26–35, for this group.   2. *ibid.*, i, 37–41. 3. *ibid.*, i, 42–4.

with the Western enema, except that it is done without the can and the tube apparatus using the pressure of the atmosphere, but applies water pressure direct. It is done by first standing on the toes, or rather on the balls of the feet, then squatting down on the heels,[1] this being done in water deep enough to reach the navel, and then admitting and expelling water by alternate dilation and contraction of the anal sphincter-muscle. This is said to be a help in cases of urinary trouble, wind, and similar internal disorders.

In the dry method – which is done not in water but on the ground, of course – one sits with both legs straight out in front, but not touching each other and with the forehead bent down between the knees (as near as possible) and the hands holding the toes. In this position, give a downward pressure to the bowels and slowly dilate and contract the sphincter-muscle of the anus as in the wet method. The benefits of both methods are stated to be the same.[2]

The *neti-yoga* (nostril cleaning) is done with a fine thread, a span in length,[3] put into one of the nostrils and sniffed up until the end can be pulled out through the mouth, through which, after a little movement, it is withdrawn. Besides removing nasal secretions, this also is credited with promoting clairvoyance.[4]

The *laulikī-yoga* (loosening the abdominal contents) is done by moving the belly with vigorous energy from side to side.

The *trātaka* (clearing the vision) consists of looking at a small object without shutting and opening the eyes (blinking), until tears begin to fall. There is no suggestion of staring; there is only looking. One must emphasize this, because there should be no strain or tenseness, and the object should be at a distance which involves no conscious focusing. I believe the best form of this exercise to be that in which the small object is on a level with the eyes and at a distance of about twenty feet. The idea is that there should

1. The *utkatāsana*. 2. *Gheranda Sanhitā*, i, 45–9.
3. A long span, one must say, a foot or more in length.
4. *ibid.*, i, 50, 51.

be no movement of the eyes, which is arranged for by having an object small enough to prevent looking at various parts of it, and by avoiding winking. To stare or strain would be injurious, but this proper kind of looking is not only considered to be beneficial to the eyes and conducive to clairvoyance, but also as leading to what is called the *shāmbhavī mudrā*. It may be explained here that *shāmbhavī* means related to Shiva, and Shiva is that aspect of the divine power which is concerned with lifting men up from their bondage to body and mind so that they may come to know the spirit by direct perception.

The *mudrā* is described as looking between the eyes or eyebrows, as, for example, in the *Bhagavad Gītā* (v, 27–8) where it says:

Having put the external contacts outside and (having made) the gaze even between the eyebrows, (and) having made equal the in and out breaths travelling within the nose, (and) with senses, *manas* and *buddhi* controlled, the aspirant (*muni*), with liberation (*moksha*) as his chief aim, his desire, fear and anger being gone – it is even he who is always free (*mukta*).

Further to this, it is explained that 'when by the occurrence of great fortunateness Kundalinī has become awake, and joined with the Self (*ātmā*) it goes out through the passage-way between the eyes, and enjoys itself in "the royal road".'[1] The yogi, however, becomes conscious of his subtle body thus going out, as a result of his practice of *shāmbhavī mudrā*, which has already been explained as his calm, steady looking between the eyebrows. The term 'royal road' refers to what is called travelling in the subtle body.

Another development from the *shāmbhavī mudrā* occurs when the yogi, while performing the act, proceeds to the direct perception of the Self (*ātmā*), and having seen Brahman in the point (*bindu*), he fixes his mind (*manas*) there. The aim in this case is to enter into deep contemplation (*samādhi*), not to travel in the subtle body, and this the yogi does by having the *ātmā* in the midst of the ether and the

1. *ibid.*, vi, 18, 19.

ether in the *ātmā*. The ether could also be translated space or void.[1] Because of this, and the astral travelling, the *shāmbhavī mudrā* is sometimes called the sky-walking or void-walking (*khecharī*).[2]

The *Gheranda Sanhitā* states that the practice is such that 'looking between the eyes one looks at the delightful Self (*ātmārāma*)'.[3] *Ārāma* is in ordinary usage a pleasure-garden, something delightfully peaceful to contemplate. We must give such a feeling-tone to the word here. This has to be a most peaceful kind of looking. This is the way in which one realizes Brahman as Self. All this refers, of course, to meditation and contemplation, in which with the eyes shut one sees the object as if between the eyebrows. In all such looking there must be 'attention without tension', for which a little physical *trātaka* can well be a preparation. Again it must be said, beware, even in this looking with the eyes closed, of straining the eyes.

In connexion with this practice of *trātaka* various eye exercises are often recommended which are aimed chiefly at the steadiness of the eye and its continuity (not jumping) when in motion. If material steadiness is successfully attained, and felt, the inward-looking can have steadiness with the aid of the same feeling, and so while the exercises are good for the eyes they are also good for the 'sight' of the mind. A very good set of these exercises is the following: (1) Sit at the end of a room and look at the far wall. Without moving the head let the eye travel along the horizontal lines where the floor and the ceiling meet, then diagonally from corner to corner, then round the outline of the wall, first one way, then the other – all slowly and without jumping, which is by no means an easy matter. (2) Looking at one fixed point move the head up and down, and from side to side and round and round. (3) Holding the tips of the index fingers of both hands together on a level with the eyes and at reading distance from them, observe the point of junction. Then look 'through' that junction into the far distance,

1. *ibid.*, vii, 7, 8.   2. *Mandala Brāhmana Upanishad*, ii, 18.
3. *Gheranda Sanhitā*, iii, 64.

and now you will notice a third finger between the other two, which will disappear when you look closely at the junction and will appear again as your vision extends to the distance. Try to travel from near to far and back several times slowly. All this without tension of eye or mind.

The famous Maharshi Ramana, of South India, who died a few years ago, was famous for his calm steadiness of vision, and also for his constant teaching of the steadiness of the 'I' looking at the 'I'.

We come now to the last of the group of six cleansings, called 'clearing the skull' (*kapālabhāti*). This is given as of three kinds, described as processes (*a*) of air and (*b* and *c*) of water.

In (*a*) we have simply the drawing-in of air through the left nostril and its expulsion through the right, followed by the reverse process. It is specially specified that indrawing (*pūraka*) and outbreathing (*rechaka*) must be done without any forcefulness, and that it is done to promote health, in form of removal of faults of phlegm.

In (*b*) water is drawn in through the nostrils and slowly sent out through the mouth, while in (*c*) the process is reversed, water being taken into the mouth and sent out through the nostrils.[1] One has seen the drinking through the nostrils sometimes being done by dipping the nose in a bowl of water and sucking the liquid in, and sometimes by using a glass and from it drinking the water in at one of the nostrils, just as one drinks by mouth. It is specially mentioned that the last two practices are conducive to ease of moving and the warding-off of old age.

Nearly all the practices we have mentioned above are described in other books also. In this connexion the *Hatha-yoga Pradīpikā* and the *Shiva Sanhitā* may be specially mentioned.

In the foregoing practices described in this chapter, purification is emphasized. We have also to take into account, however, another class of exercises named *mudrās*. Some of these have already been given in our Chapter 6, as

1. *ibid.*, i, 55–60.

they are combined with breathings or postures. We will now give a brief account of other important exercises of this kind.

The Abdominal Uplift (*Uddīyāna bandha*). Standing or sitting, draw the whole abdominal area inward and upward, a number of times. If one does it a hundred times a day the muscles will become strong and also habituated to the 'natural corset' position. At the termination of the exercises, whether the movement has been repeated many times or only a few, one should cease with the indrawn and lifted position. No doubt, while attending to other duties the muscles will fall down again, but one must not give a voluntary assent to this position.

While doing breathing exercises, says the *Yogakundalī Upanishad*, one should perform the abdominal uplift at the end of a breath-holding (*kumbhaka*), just at the beginning of the outbreathing (*rechaka*). It is also, however, a good practice to set up the position or hold (*bandha*) before starting an exercise in deep breathing, and retain it throughout the whole exercise. This prevents deep breathing from being over-done, to the detriment of the abdominal area.

The *uddīyāna* is also one of those exercises which can be done in bed, and is then useful before the relaxation which is conducive to good sleep.

With a little practice combined with thoughtful attention it will be found that one can perform the backward and upward action of the *uddīyāna* towards the right side or towards the left side. This is a useful variant of the abdominal uplift. A further practice is to uplift the right and left sides at the same time; this leaves a ridge in the centre, and is called *nauli*. By a combination of the movements one after the other it is possible to give the appearance that the whole abdominal contents are in rotation.

A practical question is raised among Western people, and especially women, in connexion with this exercise: should corsets or strong elastic girdles be used or not? This is a difficult question. The answer must surely vary, as it depends on the individual. If the belt is not something to lean against, but is for the most part a reminder of proper posture in the midst of the unbalanced movements of factory work or the slumping condition of sedentary occupation or the irregularities of housework, it can no doubt be very good. Whether corseted or girdled, however, the wearer should remember that the abdominal uplift can and should be done, when opportunity is offered, while wearing the garment and not only when it is off. One must not forget public morale also, for if everybody went about carelessly in such matters, we might in time come to take it for granted that the standard and expected shape of the human torso resembles that of a pear. Such a collapse of morale should be avoided at all costs.

While on the subject of posture we may bring in the question of posture of movement, which means mainly in walking. The yoga books stress uprightness in sitting so much that we assume that the teachers took it for granted that in walking their pupils would follow the same behest. It is here that the uprightness of the neck needs special attention. If the back of the neck is kept back, especially at its lower end, the shoulders are unlikely to slump, and better balance with better breathing will automatically ensue. Balance is the watchword, of course, not stiffness.

Related to the Abdominal Uplift is the Act of Inversion (*Viparītakaraṇī*), the reversal of the 'sun' and the 'moon'. It is said that the 'moon' resides at the root of the palate and the 'sun' at the root of the navel, and that the nectar (*amrita*) from the moon is thus absorbed by the sun. This refers perhaps to the tendency for the powers of the higher centres to be used by the lower in the ordinary course of life. We know that man is more prone to gluttony and sensuality than any animal because he uses his mind-power to intensify and prolong them, and to enjoy them frequently, and uses his imagination to engineer their increase.[1] It is suggested that the upright posture of man may cause some bodily pressure

1. By using cooking techniques, for example, to stimulate the pleasures of taste, which some of the Romans used to increase still more by going

which promotes or sustains or habituates this tendency to craving, and that occasional resort to the upside-down position may be of benefit as an exercise.

The exercise in this case takes the form of elevating the legs in the air while assuming a shoulder-stand. *Gheranda* states that the regular practice of this exercise or attitude (*mudrā*) delays old age and death. The position is reached by lying on the back and raising the legs and the body vertically, with the elbows on the ground and the hands supporting the body near the waist. The chin is, of course, bent in close to the chest.[1] In this position simple deep breathing exercises may be done. In raising and lowering the legs one bends the knees to decrease leverage. When regarded as a posture this is also called *sarvāngāsana* (posture of all limbs) and will be found so listed in our last chapter. Some, when doing this exercise, do not assume so vertical a position, but with the hands on the buttocks allow the back some slope. The head stand (*shīrshāsana*) is also akin to this exercise. All these positions are considered especially good in connexion with constipation, asthma, sexual weakness, etc.

There is a further addition to the head stand in which the palms of the hands are put flat on the ground and the arms are straightened, so that one stands on the hands instead of on the head. This is called the *Vajrolī Mudrā* (Thunderbolt Gesture or Exercise).[2]

A breathing practice called Bee or Beetle Drone (*bhrāmarī*), which is intended to lead on to an inner experience, is given in several of the *hatha-yoga* books. This does not mean making a sound but hearing inner sounds, when the breath is standing still in *kumbhaka*. It is to be done at

out and tickling the throat in order to vomit after fullness, after which they would return to the dining-room to eat again; or by employing birth-control and stimulating pictures and literature to serve the cult of sensuality and sexuality for the sake of pleasure without responsibility or regard for natural law.

1. See *Gheranda Sanhitā*, iii, 33–6, and *Shiva Sanhitā*, iv, 45.

2. A particularly good modern explanation of these two stands is given in Devi, Indra, *Forever Young; Forever Healthy.*

night, when all around is quiet. As *Gheranda* puts it in verse:

> When half of the night has gone
> And the sounds of living things have ceased,
> With hands over the ears
> Filling and holding of the breath should be done.
> Then one should hear
> In the ear on the right
> The sound beautiful, internal –
> First that of crickets,
> Then the delicate reed-pipe.
> Then such as the rumble of the rain-cloud,
> And bells,
> And gongs,
> And various kinds of drums.[1]

The hearing of these sounds – and similar but different sounds are cited in various accounts – is not an end in itself, but only a mode of inward attention to still the outward curiosity of the senses and outward-going tendencies of mental drift. When the practice becomes successful on account of regularity, the last of all the sounds is heard – that from the heart, called the unstruck (*anāhata*) sound in contrast to the previous sounds which have died away and been replaced by this.

The principle is that all attentiveness begins in a starting-point, and then proceeds from the coarse to the subtle, and from the subtle to the as yet unknown – the experience *within* the consciousness. The sounds are not in themselves of value. Therefore it is next said that in the sound (*shabda*) of the heart there is a resonance (*dhwani*), in that there is a light (*jyotis*) and in that there is the mind (*manas*). Then, when mind itself disappears (one is no longer thinking of it) there is the veritable supreme place (or rather standing-place) of Vishnu, the very heart and sustaining principle of conscious life.[2]

The educated Hindus like the very delicate music of the *vīnā*, on which the classical compositions sound almost spiritual, being so delicate and fine. Although so light,

1. *Gheranda Sanhitā*, v, 78–80.   2. *ibid.*, v, 81, 82.

the sound carries to a large audience most surprisingly, probably partly because the audience is always very quiet and attentive – one may say more than attentive, absorbed. I remember well an occasion on which I had been to such a recital with an Indian friend. As we walked together on the way home we conversed a little. He was speaking of the wonder of the music, and then said, 'While you are listening, you just can't think of anything at all.'

Those words describe its character very well. Common music stirs or soothes the blood or the nerves, or it tells a story and reminds us of some pleasing and peaceful scene or action, but here there was nothing but music – 'music music-born', as Emerson might have put it. Such is the conception of the *anāhatā* sounds. They are understood to be spiritual sounds, to be tasted as such.

Such a process as the *bhrāmarī* is usually called a *hatha-yoga* meditation. The *rāja-yogī* proper will proceed not by intentness on sounds or other outward things, but directly to his goal, using objects only as symbols of meaning, and going through meanings to the super-knowledge which brings him to his goal.

Gheranda comes near to this when he gives the fainting (*mūrchā*) method of *hatha-yoga* meditation. This is done by assuming a comfortable fill of breath (*kumbhaka*), after which, the mind being between the eyebrows, there is a pleasantly obtained fainting of the mind (*manas*) away from all objects. Then is born a great joy on account of the union of the mind with the real Self (*ātmā*).[1] The 'fainting', it must be noticed, is of the mind, not of the body. It swoons, as it were, with joy.

We may now turn to the question of sense-control (*pratyā-hāra*) which is mentioned after the *mudrās*, and is intended to produce bodily calmness. It is also one of Patanjali's set of eight 'limbs' (*angas*) of yoga.

On this subject Patanjali's aphorisms read:

There is withdrawal of the senses (*pratyāhāra*) when they are

1. *ibid.*, v, 83.

detached from their own proper business and are imitating, as it were, the nature of the mind (*chitta*).

From that comes complete obedience of the senses.[1]

It is well known that many things are constantly coming within the range of the senses without being noticed. Minor matters we do not notice at all. I asked a friend what was the colour of his bedroom walls, and he did not know. We cannot, in fact, pay attention to very much at any time, and when we are engaged in reading a book or thinking about something we may notice nothing at all of what is around us. I saw one motorist drive his car slap into another on an unfrequented road; he told me afterwards that he had not seen it at all until the collision occurred. He was, it seems, thinking of something else.

The aim of the yogi in this connexion is to be able not merely to withdraw attention at will from the messages coming in through the senses, but something much more – to be able to command the senses and tell them when and in what particulars to operate. This is analogous to the command of the limbs, whereby we can tell the legs, for example, when to walk and when not to walk. There is in this proposition of withdrawal (*pratyāhāra*) a fine point of possible difference of opinion, but Patanjali is quite clear in saying that the senses are detached from their own proper or regular function and that they come under complete obedience. This is a voluntary operation of what occurs involuntarily when we are intent upon something, whether an object or a thought.

As an example I may mention a friend of mine whose wife has some heart trouble which occasionally, not often, wakens her in the night. He and she sleep on separate beds against opposite walls of the room. Their bedroom window is on the ground floor and on a fairly main road where there is traffic early and late. My friend is a good sleeper through all this, but at the slightest cough or groan from his wife he is alert and up to help her. The senses are apparently awake

1. *Yoga Sūtras*, ii, 54, 55.

to certain sounds and not to others unless there is something abnormally strong or violent. Similar is the instruction that we can give to the senses before sleeping to wake us at a prescribed time. The idea is that just as we can tell the limbs to be quiet, so we can tell the senses. One could say to the senses, 'I am about to do fifteen minutes' meditation, so be quiet and do not pay attention to anything except if the house is on fire, and call me at the stroke of nine o'clock.'

There is also another aspect of the matter. During the meditation we may wish the senses to present us with pictures of the object chosen, if it is an objective (*samprajnāta*) meditation. This includes all the appropriate senses. If there is a flower, for example, we should have a good visualization of it. There should also be the scent, the feel of the texture of the petals, etc. Really, we only know objects when their messages are within the mind, and in many cases we wish to go over experiences which have been all too fleeting. It is significant that so often when we endeavour to reproduce them the pictures are very poor, and yet during dreams they are as clear as possible.

In this we have an instance of the senses desisting from their usual business and imitating, as it were, what is in the mind. All these things are made more perfect by deliberate practice.

CHAPTER 8

THE LATENT BODY-POWER OF YOGA

WE come now to a group of yoga practices entitled the *laya-yoga*. It is stated that there resides a 'force' latent or almost latent in the average human being, at or near the base of the spine. This is called Kundalinī, a word which means coiled up.

The use of the word force to describe the Kundalinī is, however, misleading, if we are to use the word at all carefully or scientifically. In yoga literature it is spoken of as a goddess (*devī*). The superior reader may smile at this, until he has understood why this word is used in preference to 'force'.

The explanation is that we are dealing with three kinds of realities and influences: (1) Matter, which tends to equilibrium (the articles of furniture in our rooms do not suddenly get up and move into different places or molest one another); (2) physical force, which 'runs down', or serves matter in the adjustment of disturbed equilibrium or to relieve a condition of strain (water will run downhill, or hot air will rise in the atmosphere – there are innumerable effects of physical and chemical forces); and (3) *something else* that serves consciousness in the body by developing and maintaining organs for its expression and enjoyment. All these three are 'material facts' and should be called by different names. The third, being neither matter (in the ordinary sense) nor force (in the ordinary sense) must be called by another name and the most suitable is something 'divine'.[1]

A definition of matter which will satisfy is 'that *principle*

1. The idea of a spiritual element in the material event seems akin to the Christian idea of the Holy Ghost as being with us always in a small degree, even materially, and capable of inspiring a divine enhancement of material faculty, resulting in 'miracles', as spoken of in the upper chamber where the disciples met at Pentecost.

in Nature by which the past is carried into the present'. The mind may be similarly defined as 'that principle in Nature by which the future is brought into the present'. In the latter case the idea is that if one plans to do something to-morrow one is planning the future, and when tomorrow comes we find that planned occurrence actually taking place. But there has to be a third principle, in which mind and matter can meet, which is life. Living can indeed be defined as the meeting of mind and matter. There is thus a line of living, on which the meeting is life. The unphilosophic man, if asked what his life is, says, 'It is getting up in the morning, dressing myself, having breakfast, going to my office . . .' and that is true, because in every moment there is the meeting of matter and mind, the past and the future, and that so-called present moment is a unit of time which is triple – a *tryanuka*, as the old philosophers called it.

I hope it is not too much to ask of the Western reader to bear with me while I try to explain the idea of the presence of the divine in three ways. The three ways are: (1) in the body, (2) in the mind, and (3) above both.

When it is said that God is present always and everywhere, people usually think of a benevolent loving father looking down and intervening when it seems good and proper to him. That is God as a great and good mind and will, even to the extent of being all-powerful. Some add to this the idea that he does these acts of goodness and power through his angels as agents or, shall we say, since the angels have nothing to do but serve God, as more than agents – positive expressions of himself? In this case the angels are varieties of his actual presence.

The next point is that people respond variously to these 'angels', sometimes being so crass as not to respond at all. This being so, it is part of the path of common sense and wisdom to try to pay attention to them. When on any occasion the angel's good advice and/or help is received, there is gratitude, and gratitude begets love, and love begets worship, which is essentially service. Then worship begets closer contact and receptiveness, and these beget union with God in the department or activity of being concerned in the given case.

If we say that all is under law, and laws are good for us because even the laws of Nature foster our intelligence and conscious growth, then those laws are really Laws, that is angels or expressions of the presence of God, such angels[1] being completely steady and continuous in the performance of their duties. Surely no one expects matter to be the cause of itself, and if they do they are proposing that such matter is different from every manifestation of matter – which has cause – that is, different from everything we know, and furthermore, endowed with the power or nature of being the one thing which is the cause of everything else. It is better, is it not, to assume that there is something beyond both matter and mind, especially since mind itself is subservient to law, and though it is clever in creativeness can work only in obedience to laws within and outside itself?

Well, then, these angels *are* parts of God, who is one in the midst of his own variousness, inasmuch as they have no other being, or nature, or business, and are in no conceivable way separate from him.

Such are the thoughts – in different degrees of depth – which have caused the worshippers of the deities in all the *chakras* (or subtle centres in the body) to pay their devotions to the 'gods' and 'goddesses' or divinities in each, and to Kundalini, regarded as the mother of them all.

The yogis, and Hindus generally, prefer to call this power that vitalizes all the centres a goddess rather than a god, because they think of all the material side of things as feminine and receptive, while the mind side is regarded as masculine. Man gives the germ to woman and she cherishes and develops it and produces the child. In India even the great gods cannot do material things; their wives do everything for them. The goddess principle thus came to be called the *shakti*, the power. Woman cherishes things and

1. Such 'angels' must not be anthropomorphized, of course. There is matter, energy, and law in nature, and law is the presence of the divine, which is good for us, and is to be respected and rightly used.

thus makes the home, and promotes material continuity. The big house called Nature has matters, energies, and laws.

The word *shakti* means literally ability. It has frequently been translated as power. In this conception there is a challenge to the Western theory of material causation in which only matter and force are taken into consideration. Matter and force are both mechanical, but this 'third thing' provides for growth or evolution, which in turn, however, is regarded as taking place by purification, which allows more and more of the divine fullness to be experienced and expressed.

This mother-power in the body is regarded as usually latent, as regards its third or highest or divine character. The earth-power works in a routine way through the *nādīs* or channels outside the spine, on the left and on the right (called *idā* and *pingalā*) but not usually in the central channel, the fine *chitrinī*.

It has now to be aroused or awakened, and will then go up the spine on a journey to the other end of it, the brain. In doing so, it will pass through, and perhaps linger in, six stations, called *chakras* (wheels), or *padmas* (lotuses) – terms derived from their appearance. These *chakras* are, however, very fine (*sūkshma*). They are, in fact, not threaded upon the coarse spine which we know by our physical senses of sight and touch, but upon a very fine channel (a *nādī*) within it.

The descriptions, which are numerous, state that within the spinal cord, generally taken to be what is called *sushumnā* in the yoga books, there is a finer cord named *vajra*, and within that again a still finer, named *chitrinī*, on which the six *chakras* are threaded, and up which the Kundalinī goes.

The practices involved in awakening the Kundalinī and taking it or guiding it, or allowing it to go, into or through the six *chakras* and to its goal beyond them in the upper part of the head, are called the *laya-yoga*. They are described mainly in two classes of yoga literature – the *hatha-yoga* books, and the *tāntric* books. The former describe what functions in the body are stimulated by the temporary residence of

Kundalinī in the several *chakras*; the latter give very minute and full directions as to the kind of concentration and meditation and worship which should be carried on within each of them. It is indeed from the precision of these instructions that the term *tāntric* arises, the general idea of a *tantra* being a set of guiding lines such, for example, as the long threads or warp on which a cloth is woven, or such as the railroad lines on which a train runs. There is a quite well-established course for Kundalinī.

Before proceeding to describe these yogas, it will be well to examine the idea of latency. In modern physical science we are familiar with the idea of potential energy. This is not just nothing – potential in the sense of 'possible'. It implies an interior causation, an involvement of built-in energies which are balancing one another so that no action takes place. The most familiar illustration of this is an object lifted from the floor and placed just on the edge of a table. It is conceived that the energy expended in lifting it is now residing in it in a latent or inactive condition, and this is proved by the fact that if the object is now pushed off the edge of the table it will give out in falling the same amount of energy as was put into it in the lifting of it. The force in the atom, appearing when the atom is 'split', is another example of latent energy, it being presumed or surmised that somehow in the workshop of Nature the great force or rather balance of forces in the atom has been packed in there in the course of the gradual production of what we call the physical world, the world of the senses.

We have now, however, to conceive of coiled-up potential energy, or curved latency. We are familiar in modern science with the conceptions of static and dynamic inertia. If a billiard ball is at rest on the table, it will remain so for ever unless disturbed by something else. If it is moving along it will continue so moving in the same straight line for ever unless impeded by something else. Therefore it is possible to predict where the ball will go. If a straight line is prolonged you can predict where it will go. But if a curved line is prolonged you cannot predict where it will go, because a curve is *all curve* and there is no straightness at all in it, not even in the smallest piece of it. And as there is no straightness at all in it, not even in the smallest piece of it, and as there is an endless variety of curvatures, but only one straightness, we cannot predict where the curve will go.

So I will venture to say that the picture of Kundalinī as a coiled-up force suggests that it is a life-force, or curved inertia. Living forms, whether plant or animal, are characterized by curves. We have to note that the Kundalinī energy in the body is not stated to be sucked into the body from outside it, but is described as welling up from within. We could perhaps, for convenience, think of it by the illustration or analogy of a new storage battery; when the energy is released it proceeds along the lines provided, that is up the *Chitrinī* canal (or *nādī*), and into or through the *chakras* in their established order or sequence.

It is not imagined that the *chakras* are themselves sources of energy, though each one is concerned with the functions of its part or section of the body.[1] They are like machines.

In considering the variety of the *chakras*, the simile of a prism and spectrum may again help us to picture the variety of functions and effects of the force operating through such a set of centres. Or we may regard them as differently coloured bulbs or different electrical machines or motors on a circuit.

The *laya-yoga* practices are to be regarded as a sort of voluntary evolution of bodily powers beyond the normal capacity or range. As the sensitive spot on the skin of a very primitive organism gradually developed by the combination of the creature and its environment, or desire and circumstances, into the complexity and capacity of an eye, so our present senses are regarded as mere sensitive spots as com-

1. They have been said to correspond to the cervical (neck) region of seven vertebrae (*vishuddha*); the dorsal (upper back) region of twelve vertebrae (*anāhata*); the lumbar (lower back or waist) region of five vertebrae (*manipūraka*); the sacral region of five vertebrae (*swādhish-thāna*); and the coccygeal region of four imperfect vertebrae (*mūlādhāra*). See *Kundalini Yoga* by Shivanada, and *The Mysterious Kundalini* by Vasant Rele.

pared with what can be developed by the *laya-yoga*. In such a voluntary evolution of a pre-established pattern (like seed and tree) there is the difference between the stem of the lotus groping upward through the water, and the blossoming of the lotus when it reaches the air and the sunshine, and, in the theory of *laya-yoga*, when the Kundalinī reaches the 'thousand-petalled lotus' (*sahasrāra chakra*) after passing through the six *chakras* and completing her journey to the top of the head, she (the earth-power or body-power – the body's ability to be body – being regarded as feminine) joins with her spiritual spouse (receives the spiritual sunshine) and blossoms, giving new radiance to all the *chakras* when she returns through them back to her own home at the base of the spine. The machinery of the body now flowers, as it were, into new beauty and power on account of its new dedication to the service of the spiritual will, the sublimated or enlightened will-to-live which is the will-to-fulfilment. Therefore, before yoga the bodily functions were only a preparing, but now the true man is born and every function is sanctified and enhanced by the new service.

The *rāja-yogīs* whom I have known do not quite approve the methods of the *laya-yogīs*, which we will presently describe, which consist of external and mental means to awaken Kundalinī so that she starts up hissing like a sleeping snake which has been disturbed by a poking stick. They regard it as if a mother were to pull or slap the legs of a child to induce it to walk, or as if a gardener were to use external force on the budding petals of a rose to induce it to open. They say that when there is high meditation – the endeavour to understand, feel, and realize the higher and finer things – Kundalinī rises automatically and culminates from time to time in the thrill of ecstatic intuition and the subsequent permanent benefits to the *chakras*, which can best be left to take care of themselves. Patanjali makes no mention of spinal channels and *chakras*, nor of Kundalinī.

It will be seen that herein lies the function of worship or devotion. In the West people are often devoted to an ideal

– beauty, truth, goodness, etc. But in *laya-yoga* devotion is thus not mere pious sentiment, as is sometimes thought, but is something definite, which brings about the building grace of Kundalinī. The same principle has operated through the course of biological evolution – the evolving organisms have never formulated or designed a living organ for themselves, but they have aspired to live (to increase their living and conscious experience) in various environments, and Kundalinī has done the rest. We cannot say that any application of force or of idea by us has produced our limbs; they have come as a grace in response to our will to live, which contains also the will-to-live-more, which is the instinctive worship of life.

If it is argued (as some Tāntrists have done) that one should have the full and most enhanced bodily enjoyments along with one's spiritual gains, and should not hold that spiritual progress involves the abandonment of bodily pleasures, the answer of the *raja-yogī* is that this is true to the extent that along with purification and high insight there naturally come enhanced sensitiveness and enjoyment in the body, but, as all this life is only a schooling for the spiritual life, when the spiritual life becomes known, all these pleasures are as nothing compared with the joy of that self-realization, and so, as Patanjali puts it, 'To the enlightened all (this) is misery',[1] only, of course, we must emphasize the enlightenment and not think that making oneself miserable is a means to that end. And this is consistent with the *rāja-yoga* method of non-pursuit of enjoyment, and intentness upon the open mind and heart, leading to unveiled spiritual perception. One who understands this and so does not eat for the pleasures of taste will in the course of eating for health obtain more pleasure of taste than can be obtained by the pursuit of gustatory pleasure.

Before we come to the listing of the *chakras* and the description of worship in them, it seems necessary to speak of the gods and goddesses who are regarded as resident in them.

1. *Yoga Sūtras*, ii, 15.

Why should natural forces or functions be pictured in these very personal terms? The answer is that as long as you cannot know the roots and sources and axes (so to speak) which have determined the specification of the classifiable groups and varieties of conscious experience it is better to speak of them in terms of personal life than in terms of lifeless matter and force. If anyone protests against the anthropomorphic description of God and gods, he must also take care not to fall into a 'mineralomorphic' one, in which he would find himself talking about 'forces' and 'lights' and 'voids'.

The average worshipper of personalized gods is well aware that his pictures and statues are only a makeshift, a sort of language, which he often regards, however, as superior to word-language. Take, for example, the three great gods: Shiva is only God's will or purpose, Vishnu God's love or kindness, and Brahmā God's materially creative presence. And even this will, love, and thought are only regarded as expressions or manifestations of the one divine Reality (*sat*), Consciousness (*chit*), and Joy (*ānanda*), which are beyond mind.

To call these ultimate powers will, love, and thought is to continue the same mistake – mind-anthropomorphism. The conception of gods contains something more than matter and mind, but applied to these two. There is in fact one 'school' of thought which holds that when a human being has perfected his intelligence and/or his love and/or his will, he still needs some further schooling in the use of these faculties under the divine guidance. Thus, to compare it with Christian thought, man's perfect intelligence is not enough, for it needs the infusion of the Holy Ghost, man's perfect love is not enough, for it needs the infusion of the Christ, and man's perfect will is not enough, for it needs the infusion of the divine Presence. And all this, of course, in the same old world, but a world seen full of new significance.

Not only in the pictured or imagined contents of the *chakras* are there these various gods, but in the homes of the people one may constantly find such pictures on the walls. It is then very instructive to find that in conversation these gods are alluded to as 'the pictured ones' (*nilimpas*). They are indescribable in terms of, or in comparison with, any of the contents of this world of ours or of our mind, so they are something that is 'pictured', not known. And 'something' here has to be used with caution, for the reality can only be spoken of as 'that', not as 'this'. Matter is not a self-existent, self-producing, and self-maintaining reality, existing and eternal in its own right and to be taken for granted as such, any more than mind is; nevertheless, the world is not just a heap of unclassified oddments, but everywhere there is law, order, classification, and intelligibility, which mind as well as matter has to acknowledge and obey as subordinate. The gods represent these 'laws beyond mind', and their pictures serve as mental foci for concentration and meditation and that contemplation (*samādhi*) in which the mind and all its works are transcended and the consciousness of man communes with the laws, to which it is fundamentally akin.

Let us now proceed to a description of the *chakras*, and the meditations or, rather, worship in them.

The six *chakras* (wheels) or *padmas* (lotuses), counting downwards along the spine, are listed as:

1. *Ājnā:* between the eyebrows.
2. *Vishuddha:* at the throat.
3. *Anāhata:* at the heart.
4. *Manipūraka:* at the navel.
5. *Swādhishthāna:* at the genitals.
6. *Mūlādhāra:* at the base of spine, between the anus and the genitals.

We may, for convenience, call them the eyebrow centre, the throat centre, the heart centre, the navel centre, the pelvic centre, and the basal centre. It is to be understood, however, that they are very subtle organs, threaded on the very fine *chitrinī* canal within the spinal cord, and that the regions of operation or influence extend over considerable areas of the body. They are the media of communication between the mind and the body, so just as the sense organs are not the senses, so are the nerve-plexus or ganglia in the body not the sources of nervous impulses arising from thought, but merely instruments for them.

Some writers[1] have gone so far as to identify the *chakras* with the nerve-plexuses – in order, the cavernous, the pharyngeal, the cardiac, the epigastric, the hypogastric, and the pelvic. Others hold that there is merely 'some connexion' between these plexuses and the *chakras*, respectively. But the yogis in general ignore the bodily details – as has been already explained – and leave the centres to attend to any details of their work, just as we ignore the nerves and muscles of the legs when walking. But it is held by all the *hatha-yogis* and *tāntrikas* that thought upon or within the *chakras*, stimulates or quietens them, as the case may be, and this viewpoint lies behind their practices of meditation and worship within the *chakras*.

This belief in the influence of thought is borne out by general experience, for when very intent upon listening to something we do instinctively 'put our consciousness in the ears', that is, concentrate our attention there. I remember too, that when, as a boy, I and others were doing Sandow's exercises for the development of the muscles, we were told to put our minds on the biceps, etc., in order to get results, and certainly not to let the mind wander away to other topics while we were making the movements. Indeed, the influence of mind on body is so well known that it barely needs mention.

It should next be noted that each lotus is pictured with petals and a centre or pericarp. The petals are given as 2 in the Eyebrow Lotus, 16 in the Throat Lotus, 12 in the Heart Lotus, 10 in the Navel Lotus, 6 in the Pelvic Lotus, and 4 in the Basal Lotus.[2]

On each of these petals a letter of the alphabet is engraved. The theory is that every letter of the Sanskrit alphabet (which is probably the most scientific in the world for phonetic arrangement) represents a basic sound, and spoken words are only compounds of these basic sounds, just

1. Particularly Dr Vasant G. Rele, in his *The Mysterious Kundalini*.
2. There are some differences in different source books. In the Heart Lotus, the *Yogakundalī Upanishad* gives 16 petals; *Dhyānabindu Upanishad* and *Shāndilya Upanishad* both give the Navel Lotus 12.

as a picture is a compound of basic and inconvertible colours. Next, sound is the basis of creative manifestation. First comes a command, which is mental, which is next expressed in an uttered sound. From sound forms arise. Also by sound forms are affected, especially the senses and sensitive forms constituting our bodies. Conversely, every movement in the world is considered to give rise to a sound, though it is often beyond the range of our ears.

This theory of sound lies behind the doctrine of *mantras*, words of power and influential chants or mutterings. Certain statements beautifully and aptly expressed are regarded as very influential, and are repeated not only for the purpose of keeping a thought before the mind, but also with the idea that the words themselves, as sounds, produce effects in line or in tune with the thoughts which are being concentrated upon. An important part of the worship conducted in the *chakras* consists of recital of *mantras*. The individual letters of the alphabet have some mantric power, but each of the *chakras* has a special fundamental one, which is therefore called its seed (*bija*) *mantra*.

We may describe the seed *mantra* of the Basic *Chakra* as typical, and then list the others. This seed *mantra* is *laṁ* (written ऌं). It is necessary to give this Sanskrit form in order to explain the pronunciation. The consonant l (which some have said looks like the claw of a crab) has on top of it a little crescent with a dot above it. Every consonant is pronounced with the short vowel a, unless some other vowel is indicated, so the main sign in this case is la. The crescent and dot on top indicate an m, prolonged, which however is not an ordinary m, in which we close the lips and then open them when enunciating the letter, but is simply the sound with the lips closed. The lips are open in saying 'la', but are closed as soon as we begin to say 'm', and in this case are not opened again, though the sound is prolonged as much as we like, and generally to the length of three syllables.[1]

---

1. Some writers have spelt this terminal sound as 'ang', it being understood that there is no sound of the g, and that the n is not as in the

The letters engraved on the petals are also each supplied with the same aftersound, and the vowel a is always short (the a in *lam* is not as in our word lamb, but like the a in America or India).

Also in considering the mantric effect of these sounds, it is to be taken into account that certain sounds have affinities with particular 'elements' (such as earth, water, fire, etc.), with particular colours, and with particular senses and parts of the body. Thus *lam* is expecially related to the earth element, the colour yellow, and the lower extremities of the body.

The seed (*bīja*) *mantras* of the six *chakras* are:

(1) The Brow Centre, *Oṁ*.
(2) The Throat Centre, *Haṁ*.
(3) The Heart Centre, *Yaṁ*.
(4) The Navel Centre, *Raṁ*.
(5) The Pelvic Centre, *Vaṁ*.
(6) The Basic Centre, *Laṁ*.

These *bīja mantras* are further depicted as riding on certain animals, except in the case of *Oṁ* in the Brow Centre. The animals give some indication of the nature of affinities of the centres and the *mantras*. The list is:

Haṁ is on a white elephant; *Yaṁ* on an antelope; *Raṁ* on a ram; *Vaṁ* on a crocodile-like fish; and *Laṁ* on another kind of elephant. These somewhat illustrate the statements that the Throat Centre is associated with the element ether (*ākāsha*) and hearing; the Heart Centre with the air element, easy movement and touch; the Navel Centre with the element fire or heat and the sense of sight; the Pelvic Centre with water and taste; and the Basic Centre with earth and smell. When meditating in a centre with the 'element-region' and 'element-faculty' or sense in mind the *bīja mantra* should be used at the beginning.

---

word 'anger'. It is another attempt to indicate the aftersound which we have described. But to write it as m seems better, or better still with a dot on top to remind the reader that there should be no definite pronunciation of m as is produced by the opening of the lips, but only the aftersound (*anuswāra*).

Along with the *bīja mantras* in the pericarps of the lotuses there are also symbolic forms which indicate the nature of the 'elements', and these have their own colours, as follows:

In the Throat Centre, a white circle.

In the Heart Centre, a smoky-blue hexagon.

In the Navel Centre, a red triangle.

In the Pelvic Centre, a white crescent.

In the Basic Centre, a yellow square.

The red triangle is inverted and has a swastika design on each side, and the yellow square has eight spears which project from the corners and the middles of the sides. Colours are also given to the petals in each lotus as follows:

The Throat Lotus has petals of a smoky-purple colour, bearing in red the vowels a, ā, i, ī, u, ū, ri, rī, li, lī, e, ai, o, au, with the aftersound m, and the eject (*visarga*) h, which last is an h at the end of a word followed by a slight breathing of the simple base of the preceding vowel.

The Heart Lotus has petals of an orange-red colour, bearing in black the consonants k, kh, g, gh, n (as in ink), ch, chh, j, jh, n (as in inch), t, and th.

The Navel Lotus has petals of a greenish colour, bearing in bright blue the consonants d, dh, n (as in into), t, th, d, dh (these four being more dental than the previous t, etc.), n (as in India), p, and ph.

The Pelvic Lotus has petals of a vermilion colour, bearing in the colour of lightning the consonants b, bh, m, y, r, and l.

The Basic Lotus has petals of a crimson colour, bearing in gold the letters v, sh (light, as in ensure), sh (heavier, as in shovel), and s. In all cases there is one letter on each petal.[1]

1. For details and coloured illustrations of these forms and colours, as well as all other information about the *chakras*, the reader is recommended to Arthur Avalon's voluminous translation and explanation of the *Shatchakra Nirūpana*, Madras (Ganesh & Co.), under the title of *The Serpent Power*. A set of very excellent coloured illustrations of the *chakras* also appears in Sri Deva Ram Sukul's *Yoga and Self-Culture*. Verbal descriptions of the *chakras* occur in numerous Sanskrit works, including *Shiva Sanhitā*, *Hatha-yoga Pradīpikā*, *Gheranda Sanhitā*, *Yoga-kundalī Upanishad*, *Dhyānabindu Upanishad*, *Shāndilya Upanishad*, *Saundarya Laharī*, etc., which do not all agree in details. There are also numerous modern books on the subject published in India, among which may be mentioned Swāmī Shivānanda's book, *The Chakras*.

From the above the reader will understand that he who meditates upon the letters, symbols, and colours in the *chakras* will have plenty to think about, and much consideration of relationships and correspondences. But now we have to add the symbols offered for devotion and worship in the several *chakras*, depicted as a god and a goddess in each. These gods and goddesses have varying numbers of heads and arms, the latter as well as other parts of the body bearing symbolic tools or weapons and offering various signs and gestures.

In the Throat Centre the god is Sadashiva, having five heads and ten arms. The hands hold a trident, a battle-axe, a sword, a thunderbolt, a fire-weapon, a cobra, a bell, a goad, and a noose, and one of them gives the sign of courage or no fear. On his body, which is smeared with ashes, he has a tiger skin, and about his neck a garland of snakes. On his forehead he wears a crescent moon, turning downwards and exuding nectar. The feminine deity in this Centre is Shākinī, who is his *shakti*, or power in the world. She is white, wears a yellow *sārī* (dress), and has four arms and five faces with three eyes each. In her hands are a bow, an arrow, a noose, and a goad.

The deities (*devatās*) in the Heart Centre are Īsha and Kākinī. Īsha – another form of Shiva – has three eyes and two arms. One hand makes the sign of granting a boon, and the other the sign of removing fear. Kākinī is also three-eyed, but has four arms, two of which give the same signs of giving a boon and dispelling fear, while the other two hands carry a noose and a skull. She is yellow in colour, and wears the skin of an antelope and many ornaments. In addition, in the middle of this Centre there is an inverted triangle in which Shiva himself is present, gold in colour and wearing as head-ornament (or crest-jewel) the crescent moon.

It must be mentioned also that just beneath the Heart Centre there is another, smaller one – a red lotus with eight petals, and therein is depicted an island of gems, containing an altar where the devotee worships his *guru* in deep meditation. This is considered one of the most beautiful descriptions of devotional meditation in all the Sanskrit literature.[1]

> Let him find in his heart a broad ocean of nectar,
>   Within it a beautiful island of gems,
> Where the sands are bright golden and sprinkled with jewels.
>   Fair trees line its shores with a myriad of blooms,
> And within it rare bushes, trees, creepers, and rushes,
>   On all sides shed fragrance most sweet to the sense.
>
> Who would taste of the sweetness of divine completeness
>   Should picture therein a most wonderful tree,
> On whose far-spreading branches grow fruit of all fancies –
>   The four mighty teachings that hold up the world.
> There the fruit and the flowers know no death and no sorrows,
>   While to them the bees hum and soft cuckoos sing.
>
> Now, under the shadow of that peaceful arbour
>   A temple of rubies most radiant is seen.
> And he who shall seek there will find on a seat rare,
>   His dearly Beloved enshrined therein.
> Let him dwell with his mind, as his teacher defines,
>   On that Divine Form, with its modes and its signs.

In the Navel Centre the two deities are Rudra and his *shakti* Lākinī. Rudra is another form of Shiva. This form looks old, and looks white – though really red – because covered with ashes. He has three eyes and the two hands give the signs for boons and fearlessness. Lākinī has three three-eyed faces and is four-armed, dark but wearing a yellow *sārī* and many ornaments. Two of her hands give the same signs; the other two carry the thunderbolt and fire-power weapons. Although having a fearsome aspect, she is entirely benevolent.

In the Pelvic Centre is the god Hari or Vishnu, of a blue colour and clothed in yellow. He is four-armed, carrying a conch, a disc, a mace, and a lotus. Special marks of his are a curl (*shrivatsa*) on the breast, taken to represent the material principle, which he lightly bears on the surface of his being, as it were, and a resplendent garland of jewels (named *kaustubha*), which has an orange-red colour, representing the souls which are part of his being as the god

1. I quote my own translation of this from the *Gheranda Sanhitā* (vi, 2–8), which appears in Wood, Ernest, *Concentration*, p. 113.

who enters (*vishati*) the world, and sustains the lives which makes it a world of the living, not of the dead.

With Vishnu in this centre is the goddess and agent (*shakti*) Rākinī, also of a blue colour. This blue colour, in the case of Vishnu, is often described as the colour of the dark rain-cloud, which is regarded in India as such a blessing when it comes to shed its life-giving rain upon the earth, vitalizing the seeds and hence sustaining all loco-motive life as well. Rākinī's blue colour is, however, des-cribed as like that of the blue lotus – a flower much admired – as she sits adorned with divine garments and holding various weapons in her hands.

In the last of the Centres, the Basal, is found the god Brahmā, the creator of the material world, in association with Indra, the deity in charge of the element ether (*ākāsha*), or skyey matter. Brahmā is represented as having four heads (some say symbolizing four directions or extensity) and four arms. In this case the goddess is Dākinī.

Enough has been said about the gods and goddesses to show that there is an almost incredible wealth of detail regarding them spread out for the meditations of the devotees, who are thus introduced to many great ideas in the fields of cosmology, philosophy, and psychology. While the mind is being thus exercised, devotion is encouraged by the contemplation of the rich variety of excellences spread out before the worshipper, who becomes more and more aware of these (in contrast to the chaos or disorder that might possibly be in the world) as his thinking puts him more and more in tune with the life-side and the divine source of things, and the awakening of Kundalinī brings him intuition and illumination beyond the range of mere thinking. It is impossible here to mention more than a fragment of the stimulating symbology given in this field by the *Shatchakra Nirūpana*,[1] and similar works.

Two things more remain to complete the story of the *chakras* – a description and account of the Brow Centre, which in important respects differs from the group of five

[1]. Translated by 'Arthur Avalon', in *The Serpent Power*.

now described, and of the *sahasrāra chakra* at the top of the head. These, with an account of Kundalini's tour will best be given in a separate chapter – our next.

We ought, however, before leaving the topic of the relation of the elements, with their *bīja mantras*, to the *chakras*, to state that there is another system of thinking about these elements and *mantras*, which allots them to sections of the body and connects a course of meditation with these. This system is perhaps best outlined in the *Yogatattva Upanishad*, briefly, as follows:

From the feet to the knees is the region of Earth, which element is four-sided and yellow, and has the letter *l*. Carry the breath with the aid of the *mantra laṁ* from the feet to the knees, contemplating Brahmā with four faces, and of a golden colour. Concentration of this kind for two hours gives more mastery over solids, and less danger from them.

From the knees to the anus is the region of Water, which is crescent-shaped, is white, and has the *mantra vaṁ*. Here the meditation is on Nārāyana, with four arms, a crown, and orange cloths. This (Vishnu) is undecaying (in contrast with the material or earthy). The benefits of the two-hour concentration are freedom from sins and mastery over liquids.

From the anus to the heart is the region of Fire. This is triangular, red, and has *raṁ* for its *bīja mantra*. Raise the breath, made resplendent by the *mantra raṁ*, along this region, contemplating Rudra, with three eyes, smeared with ashes (after the manner of yogis), and having a pleased look. Here the result will be felicity in the use of fire, and freedom from danger from that element.

From the heart to the middle of the eyebrows is the region of Air. This is hexagonal, black, and shining, with the letter *ya*. When the breath is carried along this region with the *mantra yaṁ* for two hours, with concentration on Ishwara – omniscient, with faces on all sides, the benefits of the element will be obtained.

From the eyebrows to the top of the head is the region of ether (*ākāsha*, the all pervading element). This is spherical and of a smoky-blue colour, and has the letter *ha*. Here, on raising the breath for two hours with the *mantra haṁ*, and having the vision of Sadāshiva, one gains the eight occult powers of unlimited smallness, largeness, lightness, heaviness, vision, movement, creativeness, and control. Shiva is here the Great God (Mahādeva), producing happiness, having the character of a point (*bindu*), shining like pure crystal, wearing a crescent moon on the head, with five faces, ten heads, and three eyes and a pleased expression, armed with all weapons, adorned with all ornaments and having Umā (his spouse or *shakti*) as half of his body. He, the cause of all causes is there, ready to grant favours and bestow unfailing bliss.

By practising these five meditations, it is said, the proficient yogi overcomes death, that is, he can decide when to go, and also, it is said, step out without any intervening sleep or break in conscious continuity.

The account also explains that the candidate should also practise the *mahā bandha* and the *mahā vedha* and similar exercises already given in our Chapter 7 and finally recite the *Om*, remembering that the world and life are full of threes – it is a fundamental classification in tune with the characters of the three great Agencies, Gods, or Angels.

CHAPTER 9

THE JOURNEY AND GOAL OF THE
LATENT POWER

FOR the understanding of the journey of the coiled-up power, we must first give some account of the Brow Centre, which differs from the five already described in that those are concerned with the five-fold world of the senses and the elements, while this is the *chakra* of the mind, which governs the five organs of sense and the five organs of action and at the same time serves the purpose of unifying their five-fold field and presenting the results and benefits to Kundalinī as she passes through this centre on her way to union with the pure consciousness, represented as her spouse, Shiva, residing or centred in the 'thousand-petalled lotus' at the top of the head.

It should be understood that worldly experience is not useless, but that by the clarity insisted upon by its limitation of the spread or diffusion of consciousness it enables the consciousness to waken itself more and more to the richness of its own kind and quality of being. This we have already described psychologically and illustrated by the relation between the child and the doll.

Often the books refer to the five senses, or organs for knowledge (*jnānendriyas*), 'with the mind (*manas*) as the sixth'. The five *chakras* described in our last chapter, from the Basal to the Throat Centre, are concerned with the senses from smell to hearing and the substances from 'earthy' to 'etheric'.

Now we have to consider a *chakra* (at the brow) in which the messages of the senses are woven together, whereby an intelligent understanding of the world is obtained. For example, with the eyes we 'see' a table. It is only a picture for us until we combine the sight with a memory of the feel or touch of such a thing. If we meditate upon a flower, we should be aware of its scent and the feel of its petals, not merely its appearance, in order to know its nature, what it does in relation to other things. In an elementary meditation upon a cat the students were instructed to consider: (1) 'cats I have known', (2) the qualities of a cat, as to both mind and body, (3) the parts of a cat, and (4) the classes to which it belongs, and its resemblance to and differences from other members of any such class. In this way one *puts together* all the various items one has known or can now think of about a cat. These details are not merely put together; they are positively compounded into one unitary fact or idea, which is built of its (the cat's) substance, its qualities and its actions in relation to various other things. As an example, we say that a house is one thing, showing one unitary idea; the whole embodies something not found in the parts, which might be components scattered all over the ground.[1]

Hence in the description of the Brow Centre (*ājñā chakra*) there is the statement: 'Meditation is lovely shiningness' (*Dhyānavāmaprakāsham*).[2] Meditation throws new and more light on a subject, and enhances the power of the consciousness to appreciate it.

This *chakra* is called *ājñā*, which means a command, because, it is stated, it is here that one receives the command of the spiritual teacher (*guru*). Since the object of the teacher is to enable one to replace ignorance by knowledge, his 'orders' must be understood as orders to know rather than orders to act. He provides information which the pupil left to himself may not find, and this is then built into his conception of what living properly is and should be. The *guru* guides. For this reason Buddha called himself the 'Tathāgata' – i.e. one who has gone in that manner, or has trodden the path which he describes. It is only the godness of the *guru* that is a gift, and that has to be taken by him who can.

In another way of looking at the matter, we see that this

1. For a full account of the four roads of thought, see Wood, Ernest, *Mind and Memory Training*. Occult Research Press (New York).
2. *Shatchakra Nirūpana*, 32.

manas is the commander of all our organs of action. We are always very rightly willing to make use of the habitual structures and functions of our limbs. But they are used for actions thought about and determined by the mind. Otherwise, when not being called upon for services they are supposed to remain quiet or to carry on only the necessary routines and simple responses. When one has learned to drive a car, many such responses have become habitual, but in the beginning they were commands. To be well aware of one's own mind is to be conscious of such commanding.

The Brow *Chakra* (*ājñā chakra*) is described as being beautifully white, like the moon, and having two white petals, on which the letters h and ksh are inscribed in red or in variegated colour. For this purpose *ksham* is regarded as one sound.

The deity in this *chakra* is Shiva himself, depicted in the form of a phallus (*lingam*). The mention of this symbol requires a caution to the Western reader. The thought it represents is one of great sacredness. There is in this a creative power, to be used with great forethought – not, as some casual readers may think, to be used for excited and passionate enjoyments, made further hectic by the over-stimulated imagination which modern popular literature constantly excites. The full meaning of it is that the mind is creative. It can plan new forms, design machines, invent engines. This creativeness involves two things – both the material side and the creative side are needed. In designing a clock there must be the passive and unchanging material substances and forms – wheels, levers, springs, etc. – and there must be the creative imagination. The former may well be, so to say, the womb cherishing and embodying the creative idea.

The whole universe is bifurcated in this way. The laws of arithmetic and logic apply only to the material side, and to that no longer when matter and life are joined. All the laws of arithmetic are broken when two people get married and it is soon found that 1 plus 1 equals 3.

Still another sense of the word command can be inferred

from the presence of Shiva himself in this *chakra*. In the practice of yoga the devotee strives with the mind (in the first place) to realize the meaning of Shiva, as the god who presides over the fulfilment of living. Our living is not for its own sake but as a prelude to spiritual living, which is spiritual being. Brahmā may be said to preside over the materials for living – the toyshop, may one say? Vishnu then is the caretaker of the life-side, which is mind in the fullest sense. But Shiva sees to the result. These three principles which may be compared to body, soul, and spirit, again appear in the symbols moon, sun, and fire, often mentioned in *hatha-yoga* literature.

The kind of command now being considered may well come under the heading of intuition (tuition from within) extending even to illumination. The mind is capable of receiving that, though not of creating it. First we know of something, then about it, then it; in this last, thinking ceases and the mind stands transfixed – drinking the nectar, as the poetical symbologists put it. Matter and mind are object and subject in ordinary affairs, but in this experience both are transcended.

There is, of course, always a small measure of this command in our lives. The mind is sooner or later discovered to have been all along only a servant of the inner will, which is the will not merely to live, but to adventure and even to fulfilment. 'Man never is, but always to be blest'. And yet he is blest, too, even on the road. His own 'divine discontent', did he pause to inspect it, would be found to be such a blessing.

The fact of mind-transcendence is clearly indicated in the Vedantic philosophy, where the mind, with its will and feeling and thought and imagination, is called the inner-instrument (*antahkarana*). The real pair in our lives are spirit and body; the mind is only a go-between. Indeed, the real pair are spirit and world, for the body also is only the outer instrument. In the yoga system, practices of the mind – concentration, meditation, and contemplation – are not called inmost, but only 'more within' than those of the body

– postures, breathings, sense-controls. On this, Patanjali's aphorisms are:

> The three are more within than the preceding ones. Even this (group) is an outer limb with reference to the seedless.[1]

All this has to do with Siva – the destroying will, which as it turns from one thing to another destroys or removes or abandons the old toys. 'One thing at a time and that done well' is the law of our lives, which the mind has no choice but to obey. This mind-dependency alone should prove the existence of something beyond and superior to mind.

Along with Shiva in the Brow Centre the goddess (*shakti*) Hākinī is depicted. She is shown with six heads and six arms. Four of the hands hold a book, a skull, a small two-ended drum, and a rosary. The other two give the signs of removing fear and bestowing boons. The little drum used here, and also to be seen in the hand of the dancing Shiva, needs special mention as being unfamiliar in the West. It has two drum ends with a slender or waist-like centre. A string carrying a bead is attached at the centre, so that as the hand flicks to and fro the bead strikes alternately at the ends. As before, we will not attempt to elucidate the meanings of these symbols, which would increase the size of this work too much, except to say that the skull, as in the case of similar symbols connected with Shiva, is a reminder of the passing away of all the forms; the drum indicates time, sequence, and the rhythm of manifest life (one thing after another), the rosary the benefits of concentration or continued attention and the book the value of memory.

The mind (here called *chitta*) of Hākinī is called purified (*shuddha*). In this distinction of *manas* and *chitta* one is reminded of two of the four subdivisions of the four-fold inner instrument (*antahkarana*) of the Vedantins, in which the *manas* has the business of thought while the *chitta*[2] has the business of thoughts. In other words, *manas* has the work of

1. *Yoga Sūtras*, iii, 7, 8.
2. This word should not be confused with *chit*, which means pure consciousness.

thinking, while *chitta* has recognition, memory, and the flow of associated ideas, the latter being concerned with percepts and the former with concepts, though, of course, even concepts enter the collection or museum of percepts as soon as they have been named.

In the centre of the Brow *Chakra* is an inverted triangle containing as its seed-sound (*bīja mantra*) the sign of the word Om. Om is the principal *mantra* of all the Hindu religious works. It will be described in our chapter on *mantras*. Suffice it here to say that it announces the presence of the divine.

The triangle (*trikona*) intimates here, as elsewhere, the triple nature of the one being, which is the *summum genus* of all classification, reality transcending thought, beyond the particular classes called subject and object, beyond the classification of something and nothing, beyond the conception of presence and absence, yet three-fold. The triangle in the Brow *Chakra* indicates that this three-foldness appears everywhere, and the mind should always take it into account. In the supreme reality itself, the Vedantins give the fundamental triplicity as reality (*sat*), consciousness (*chit*), and joy (*ānanda*). The Purānas (ancient legends) present the gods Shiva, Vishnu, and Brahmā. Even the philosophy of the known world (the *sānkhya*) gives its fundamental and universal substance (*prakriti*) the qualities or attributes (*gunas*) of inertia, energy, and order (*tamas, rajas*, and *sattwa*).[1]

Just as below the Heart Centre there is a minor centre for a special meditation, as described in our last chapter, so there is a minor centre (the *soma chakra*) above the *ājnā chakra*, which is stated to be concerned with ideals and good qualities of character. But we must keep to the main line in our brief account.

1. Dr Vasant Rele, mentioned in our last chapter as identifying the *chakras* with nerve plexuses of the right vagus nerve, relates the *ājnā chakra* to the naso-ciliary plexus. Usually, however, as explained before, the yogis will not accept the idea, but maintain that the *chakras* are subtle and are threaded on the channel within the spine.

The Brow *Chakra* is the last or the first of the six. But it is not the end of Kundalinī's journey. That is beyond the *ājñā chakra*, in the upper cerebral region at the top, the master centre. This is called the *sahasrāra* (thousand-petalled) *chakra*. Although called a *chakra*, it is not one of the series, because it is something quite different in character from the others. It is the goal of Kundalinī's journey, where at the end she joins her husband, Shiva, for a while. As she proceeds from the Basal Centre she passes through one *chakra* after another, and as she does so the flower (*padma*) which was previously facing downwards turns and faces upwards, it is said, then becomes cold. Psychologically, we may say, it becomes inactive or without response to appeals or stimuli coming into those centres. Before that, we could say, the attentiveness of the mind to incoming appeals of the body, with the addition of the imagination's intensification of them – that powerful spotlight of the human mind – could cause them to respond with such earth-power as they may have. This could be expressed as the flower turned downward. But when the earth-power becomes devoted to the spiritual purpose of our being (as a result of philosophy or ideals or understanding of the purpose of living, which lead to living for the sake of the inner man and even of the very Self, instead of living for pleasures of the body or pride of the mind), or in other words, when Kundalinī longs for her spouse Shiva, then as she goes upwards, the *chakras*, which were previously facing downwards, turn upwards, and afterwards act in response to the higher, with an obedience to the higher motives of the inner man.

We are thinking now only of occasions when there is deliberate meditation upon or rather in the centres, with that devotion to the gods and goddesses within them (aspects of the Shiva-Shakti combination) who represent the higher purposes. Such devotion (which has to be genuine, of course) changes the polarity so that the earth-power (*shakti*) can go *through* them and become entirely harmonized with the spiritual power at the top of the head.

When the meditation is over and the affairs of the world

have to be again attended to, Kundalinī retraces her path back to her residence in the Basal Centre, but does so 'having drunk of the nectar', her union with the above, and so vitalizing the centres with greater power than ever, born of and now obedient to the spirit within or above.[1] But as each meditation is only a temporary practice, it is a preparation for a later constant state in which the yogi can be entirely conscious of the spirit whatever he is doing. Kundalinī and her spouse will then be constantly united as the Being named Ardhanārīshwara, which is depicted as half male and half female, the union of Shiva and Shakti. As in other cases of exercising and meditation, the object is ultimately to produce a permanent result or condition.

The Ardhanārīshwara pictures to be seen so frequently in Hindu homes should be sufficient evidence that the Shiva and Shakti relation thought of in this religion is not a sexual idea but represents a conception of the combination of the two polarities of our conditioned existence. When we find the lingam[2] and the yoni[3] depicted, they are merely symbols of the positive and negative, or simpler forms of the figures in the combined Ardhanārīshwara. Some sects, it is true, have perverted the teaching, which was intended to spiritualize our functions, into an excuse for licentiousness, but these are few and are entirely disapproved of by almost everybody, as well as by the teaching of yoga and vedanta and most of the followers of tantra as well.

The spiritual nature of Kundalinī's journey is also shown by the teaching that there are three knots (*granthis*) which she has to break through – the knot of *Brahmā*, which is in the Basal Centre; the knot of Vishnu, which is in the Navel Centre; and the knot of Rudra, which is in the Throat Centre. It will thus be seen that there are three levels of con-

1. There is here an analogy to what happens when careful attention is given to something. In looking carefully at, say, a piece of red colour, and seeing it better than before, there is also developed the capacity to see red better. Thus the very consciousness is improved. And after that the consciousness will normally see better than before, without effort.

2. Male organ.

3. Female organ.

scious activity, each of which can be concerned with a change of type of activity and effectiveness. The first three centres are especially concerned with bodily effectiveness (Brahmā's overall region), the next two with the mind or soul (Vishnu's domain), and beyond those with the entry and shrine of the real man (Shiva's region). These three correspond also to the symbols of the moon (which rules the 'night'), the sun (which rules the 'day'), and fire (which is the Self ruling itself). The three groups may also be considered as dealing with the material business of life (*manas*), the benefits for the reincarnating life (*buddhi*), and the real man (*ātmā*).

All three groups are made more effective by the union of Shakti (Kundalinī) with Shiva and the consequent birthing on the return journey of the spiritually organic influence of the germinal spiritual unity in each centre – the centres being, as it were, wombs. After that the centres will have increased power and sensitiveness in their new service, instead of being centres of response and built-in impulse presenting no internal continuity but only a succession of reactions and habits. Such is the lesson of the three knots (*granthis*).

The Crown Centre (*sahasrāra chakra*) is described as having a thousand petals, marked with the entire alphabet twenty times, the whole being white and shining. In the middle of it there is a full moon, in that another triangle and in that again a Void, which is 'served in great secret by all the hosts of gods'.[1] In this we see an allusion to the state of experience beyond the mind and body, seeming a void to them. It is in this *bindu* (globule or dot; the point of the after-sound or *anuswāra*, written as a dot) that the supreme Shiva resides. There he instructs the self-controlled person with his nectar-like 'words'.

There is symbology in this dot or point. The only thing that represents the infinite is a point, and yet no one can either produce or imagine a point. We may reduce a line to less and less length an infinite number of times and yet it is still a line and not a point. At every point in the line there

1. *Shatchakra Nirūpana*, 41.

is mystery, the mystery of the straightness of the straight line and the curvature of the curved. Then there is the mystery of the freedom of the point, which is subjected to neither straightness nor curvature – neither the dead inertia of the straightness nor the living responsibility of the curve. Thus the point, represented by the *bindu*, drop or dot, does indeed indicate the abode of Shiva, the infinite. And in the sounding of the *anuswāra*, the dot on the m, there is no detectable end – no abruptness as in the sounding of other letters – but a trailing off of the sound into nothingness, whether the sounding be short or long. To think that point would be a high meditation, which would result in a conscious experience of the third estate, beyond space-measures and time-measures. We are all on the verge of it, and it only requires a conscious effort, as all other gains in consciousness have done. Kundalinī, as consciousness accepting matter and life, can join her spouse Shiva, and henceforth return to her duties afresh, being now not lonely as before (a widow, not a maiden, as the books say) but pregnant with Shiva, and always the Ardhanārīshwara, so that when you look at the Shiva you see the Shakti, and when you look at the Shakti you see the Shiva as well.

It is a considerable descent from these thoughts to a consideration of the physical ways and means of 'arousing Kundalinī' which one finds in the *hatha-yoga* and tantra literature, and also now and then among the yogis. The *rāja-yogīs*, headed by the great and classical Patanjali, will have nothing to do with these external methods. Patanjali has his '*samādhi*' – his meditation beyond thought – and he does go so far as to recommend as one of the methods towards reaching it, the recitation of *Om*, but takes care to add, 'with concentration upon its meaning'.[1] It is not that there will be no bodily change, but that the bodily change will take care of its own structuring, as has happened throughout all our evolution, in which form has always gradually conformed to serve need and desire, with due respect to the environment.

1. *Yoga Sūtras*, i, 28.

With this thought in mind, and a strong recommendation, especially to the Western reader, to be infinitely careful and gradual in any experiments he may choose to do along these lines, we will describe the methods alluded to. First, we will remember the statement that Kundalinī lies sleeping in her bulb or cave (*kanda*) at the base of the spine, where she has the nature of the *shabda-Brahman*, that is, Brahmā operating in form which is primarily sound – meaningful sound.[1]

The bulb has been described as follows:

Two fingers above the anus and two fingers below the genital organ (*medhra*) is the *kanda-mula*, in shape like a bird's egg, and four fingers' breadth in extent. The *nādīs* (nerve channels), 72,000 in number, emanate from it.[2]

The *Hathayoga Pradīpikā* adds (i, 113) that it is covered as if with a soft white piece of cloth.

As previously stated, Kundalinī sleeps here like a serpent having three and a half coils. When she is roused by suitable yogic action or meditation, she starts up, hissing, and enters the *chitrinī* channel through the gate of Brahman (*Brahma-dwāra*). This rousing, however, should not be thought of as something abnormal. In the course of time it will occur little by little quite naturally – only the practice of yoga accelerates the process.

It can of course be taken into account that in the more advanced development of every man there comes a time

---

1. This is well indicated in the *Bhagavad Gītā* (vii, 30; viii, 4) in the statement that there is an objective principle concerning the elements (*adhibhūta*) and a subjective principle concerning the life-side (*adhidaiva*), both being expressions of the oversoul (*adhyātmā*); and then another, the principle of sacrifice (*adhiyajna*), involving the interplay and mutual support of all things (fully explained in the *Gītā*, iii), this statement being followed by the words of the spirit or oversoul or *adhyātmā*: 'I here in the body am the principle of sacrifice (*adhiyajna*)', meaning that the godhead is really with us, making the interplay of body and mind, and bodies and minds possible, being the Brahman or *adhyātmā* present in the finite (thereby called *shabdabrahman* or, by the Tibetans, *fohat*), particularized in the human body as Kundalinī.

2. 'Avalon, Arthur', *The Serpent Power*, p. 324.

(in some future incarnation for the bulk of humanity) when he does take his future into his own hands, and proceeds with intention and with intuition to fulfil the last phases of human growth. This, too, should be regarded as quite natural at this stage, so that the practice of yoga is never to be looked upon as abnormal or as some special trick or dodge. Some teachers have said that it is quite an easy matter to awaken Kundalinī, but a difficult matter to take her to the higher *chakras* and all the way. Meditations, postures, breathings, and various exercises all play a part in the arousing.

The following description of a *hatha-yoga* method of arousing the Kundalinī is taken from the *Hathayoga Pradīpikā*, translated by Shrinivāsa Iyāngar:

Assuming the *padmāsana* posture and having placed the palms one upon another, fix the chin firmly upon the breast and, contemplating upon Brahma, frequently contract the anus and raise the *apāna* upwards; by similar contraction of the throat force the *prāna* downwards. By this he obtains unequalled knowledge through the favour of Kundalinī (which is roused by this process).[1]

From the Sanskrit commentary on the same the following explanation is added:

By the union of the *prāna* and the *apāna* the gastric fire is roused and the serpent Kundalinī (that lies coiled three and one half times round the *sushumnā*, closing the opening with its mouth), feels this and begins to move, straightening itself, and proceeds upwards. Then the *prāna* and the *apāna* should be forced through the hole into the Sushumnā.[2]

1. *Hathayoga Pradīpikā*, i, 48.
2. The best explanation of the three and one half coils of the sleeping Kundalinī is that there must be a triple implication or involvement of *ahankāra*, *buddhi*, and *manas* in the production of the body, with the development of a corresponding latency and potentiality. This accounts for three coils, showing some release of the power when Kundalinī penetrates the three knots (*granthis*) – i.e. the involved power corresponding to *manas* (Brahmā), *buddhi* (Vishnu), and *ahankāra* (Shiva). These gods are 'correspondences' of the three involved principles, and piercing of the *granthis* implies that the yogi has acquired some discovery of the powers of thought, feeling, and the will as independent of circumstances.

A similar method is given in the *Gheranda Sanhitā*, of which the essentials are:

Sit in the *siddhāsana*, fill the lungs with air through both nostrils, and hold it in (*kumbhaka*). Contract the rectum slowly, so as to force the down-going air (*apāna*) upwards. Kundalinī then enters the upward path. This method is called *shaktichālanī*.

An important part of it, and of the method previously mentioned, is the *ashwinī-mudrā*, described as follows:

Contract and dilate the opening of the anus again and again; this causes the awakening of the *shakti* (Kundalinī)[1].

After the *shaktichālanī* has been practised, one should complete the work, it further says, by doing the *yonimudrā*, which we may briefly describe as follows:

Sit in *siddhāsana*. Close the ears with the thumbs, the eyes with the index fingers, the nostrils with the middle fingers, the lips with the third fingers on the upper lip and the little fingers on the lower. Awaken the sleeping Kundalinī by repeating the *mantras huṁ* and *hansah*. Contemplate in the *chakras* in order, finally bringing the *shakti* to the thousand-petalled lotus. In that place contemplate the union of Shiva and Shakti in the world, with the words 'I am Brahma' realize that lake of joy.[2]

In this case it will be noticed that the air is kept within,

For example, to love one's enemies would imply such a 'freedom' of good feeling, and to be able to stand firm regardless of all dangers and pains would imply the 'freedom' of the will. In these cases love has found *itself* and the will has found *itself*. As to the half coil, it would be reasonable to see in this that part of the mind – or projection of *manas* – which is involved in the association of it with data from the material world, all the memories, etc., with which *manas* works and at the same time limits itself. Here the release of latent power would mean that where the mind was previously held to the task by being a slave to circumstances, it can now move among the circumstances and not be unduly influenced by them, as it was before. It will accept this material situation and things as they are but insist upon the paramountcy among them of reason, love, and the will, and not be dictated to by things any more. Things will no longer be in the saddle and ride this man, to use Emerson's simile, given in one of his poems.

1. *Gheranda Sanhitā*, iii, 54, 55, 82.   2. *Gheranda Sanhitā*, iii, 37–41.

after being breathed, by the fingers, but in the case quoted previously from *Hathayoga Pradīpikā*, the air is kept in by pressing the chin on the breast, which is called the *jālandhara bandha*. In the *siddha* posture (*siddhāsana*) mentioned above it will be remembered that one heel presses the anus and the other heel the root of the generative organ.

Another method presented in the *Hathayoga Pradīpikā* for the same purpose is called *mahāmudrā*. In this case:

Press the anus with the left heel. Stretch the right leg straight out, and take hold of the toes firmly with both hands. Hold the breath in at the throat (presumably by *jālandhara bandha*) and draw the air upwards. Kundalinī then becomes straight like a snake struck with a stick, and moves with the air up the central canal, while the canals on the left and right acquire the death-like state. Then very, very slowly breathe out. The exercise should be alternated by putting the right heel at the anus and stretching out the left leg.[1]

There is another method called *mahā bandha*, in which one does not stretch out the leg, but presses the anus with one ankle, and places the other foot on that thigh. Some do not use the *jālandhara bandha*, but instead press the tongue firmly against the front teeth where they join the gums.[2]

A still further extension of this method, called the *mahā vedha*, occurs when, from the same sitting position the hands are put down on the ground, the body is raised up on them, and then the buttocks are gently beaten upon the ground.[3]

Another method, still more drastic, directs:

Sit in the *vajrāsana*. Take hold of the feet firmly, and beat the *kanda* with them. Cause the Kundalinī to move by this means, and by the *bhastrikā* breath. Next the yogi should contract the region of the navel. Then, it is said, by moving the Kundalinī for about an hour and twenty minutes, she will go a little way up the *sushumnā*. Once she is in motion one should use the *bhastrikā* frequently. 'One who is celibate,

1. *Hathayoga Pradīpikā*, iii, 10–15.   2. *ibid*, iii, 19–22.
3. *ibid*., iii, 26–9.

and eats moderately of nutritious food, can obtain success in the practice of Kundalinī in forty days.[1]

Shivananda mentions a fact which for some people simplifies the whole process of Kundalinī's awakening. He says: 'While you utter the continuous sound or chant of *dīrgha pranava* (long *Om*), you will distinctly feel that the real vibration starts from the *mūlādhāra chakra*.'[2]

And now we must quote with respect to the foregoing and similar practices:

Just as the lion, the elephant, and the tiger can become tame only very gradually, so also must be treated the *vāyu* (vital air); otherwise it kills the practiser.[3]

Therefore people are generally advised to keep mainly to *rāja-yoga*, and to take up bodily practices only as far as their knowledge and wisdom and guidance permit. And to remember always that there is to be no abruptness in beginning or ending an exercise or a practice, and no continued tension in the process.

1. *ibid.*, iii, 114–22. 2. *Kundalinī Yoga*, p. 88.
3. *Hathayoga Pradīpikā*, ii, 15.

CHAPTER 10

YOGA AND VITALITY

ALL schools of yoga agree in the idea that there is in each person 'One' who sees all the other things but is not seen by them – 'some kind of self' (*kashchid swayam*), which is the 'inner Self' (*antarātman*), the 'primeval Being' (*purushah purānah*) –

By whose mere presence the organs of the body and the thinking mind and the higher intelligence all keep to their own proper forms and actions, like servants.[1]

By all such statements something indefinable is announced; really indescribable, because description involves comparisons. Just as it is impossible to say what there is when there is nirvāna, so also it is impossible to speak of this.

Yet without it, as a power of unity, there would be no organism. We see the variety of parts, and we see the harmony of their working for mutual benefit, but the unity eludes all perception, though it just has to be there. There is thus a sort of ring-master in this 'circus of many animals'.

This is the Shiva of it, while the harmony, which is goodness, is the Vishnu, and the form of the substance is the Brahmā.

In the very body is the wife of this Shiva, who is Kundalinī, who is the *vitality* of the body and of its senses and everything. On the left side and the right side of the body go the vital airs (*vāyus*) of the body – in the channel on the left called *Idā*, and in the channel on the right called *Pingalā*. These rise in the *kunda*, as does the *sushumnā* channel in the centre, and from there they branch out into the seventy-two thousand minor channels in the body. They alternate, and so resemble the symbol of the caduceus of Mercury and the symbol of the healing art of the doctors.

1. From the *Viveka Chūdāmani* of Shankarāchārya, verse 129.

There is something of a clue to the mystery of the central channel when it is said that Kundalinī goes up it when seeking Shiva. The journey takes place when there is a dedication by the yogi of all his functions, centred in all the *chakras*, to the purposes of Shiva, and the corresponding worships in all the centres, such worships being dedication of one function after another. At this point the yogi takes his living and his destiny into his own hands, instead of leaving it to the impulses of subconscious or unconscious reactions, to 'instinct'.

The books give us a list of five vital airs (*vāyus*) which are declared to have their influence in the several regions of the body. They are named *prāna*, at the heart; *apāna*, at the anus; *samāna*, at the navel; *udāna*, at the throat; and *vyāna* all over. Thus briefly states the *Garuda Purāna*.

The old teachers always very definitely described the vital airs as of five kinds, or as having five locations in the body, with different functions. The list is similarly given in the *Gheranda Sanhitā*:

Prāna moves in (the region of) the heart; *apāna* in the region of the anus; *samāna* in the area of the navel; *udāna* around the throat; *vyāna*, pervading the (entire) body.[1]

These are invariably referred to as the five principal or important *vāyus*. Five minor 'airs' are incidentally mentioned here and elsewhere, as concerned with belching and vomiting, opening and closing the eyelids, sneezing, yawning, and distributing nourishment.

The location of the five vital airs as given in the standard lists, as being associated with the centres and areas of the heart or chest, the anus, the navel, the throat, and the genitals, would indicate that they are concerned with the various functions of the body such as breathing, excretion, and digestion, as distinguished from the work of the organs of voluntary action, such as the hands, the feet, etc.

1. *Gheranda Sanhitā*, v, 61, 62. The five are also sometimes related respectively to breathing, evacuation, digestion, speech, and general energizing.

Not only in the *hatha-yoga* books are these 'vital airs' given, but in various other works. For example, in the Sānkhya philosophy, the *sūtras* of Kapila mentions them, stating that *prāna* is in the heart region, that *apāna* lies downwards from the pelvis, that *samāna* is round the umbilicus, that *udāna* is from the heart to the throat, and that *vyāna* is all over the body.

As to the last, it is not difficult to give credence to the statement that it is related to the generative function, when it is remembered that the semen draws its material from all over, and transmits something from every part of the body to the succeeding generation, and that waste of this fluid, or excessive generation of it, depletes the body all over, and on the other hand conservation of it is highly beneficial to the whole body. It appears that this is the one function of the body which does not work for the benefit of the body, but draws from it for the sake of another or others, and therefore its non-use does not harm the body but on the contrary is beneficial to it. This is at the back of the universal belief of the yogis in favour of continence and celibacy.

Many other authorities could be quoted regarding the vital airs, differing in various particulars, but presenting the same general picture. Each teacher had, and has, his own variations,[1] but in all cases it is agreed that there is no deliberate manipulation of these 'airs'. What does happen in cases of psychic healing – which takes place among *gurus* and yogis, as among modern practitioners – is that the healer gives some of his own 'vitality' by a process resembling thought-transference, or as officiating for a network

1. The elaborate list given in the *Shāndilya Upanishad*, for example, differs considerably from what may be called the standard given in many works. That the descriptions were given 'from observation' by the various old authorities on the subject is shown by the colours alloted to the vital airs. *Prāna* is generally described as of a yellow or coral colour; *apāna* as red or orange; *samāna* as green or like clouded milk; *udāna* as a pale or whitish blue; and *vyāna* as red, rosy, pale rose, or like a ray of light. The last is sometimes described as seen as a general health aura, extending a little outside the body, and appearing sturdy when there is good general health and droopy and thin when the health is poor.

of such storage. The weakness of such healing lies usually in its temporary character. The recipient of it must 'go and sin no more', or he will reproduce the old conditions which were responsible for his trouble. In any case, where there is concentration or meditation on (or better, in) centres, there is the stirring of forces, as in the case of the child learning to walk.

The feeling of health or vitality is thus not due merely to the correct working of the more or less static structures and more or less dynamic (though routine) functions of the various parts of the body, but is something *sui generis* and additional, which does not come into the body from an external place but which wells up within the body through certain centres.

So *prāna* is not the breath, but is the breath of life. And as breathing is the primary and fundamental function of the body, so is this 'electricity' required for the vitality of all the organs, and although the old teachers of yoga were not able to describe it in terms of something else already known, something other than itself (which is the basis of describing), they came as near as they could to describing it by calling it vital air or vitality. In our day we have the idea of electricity to draw upon; we can say that the body, like a battery, is well or ill charged with vitality.

Linking this whole idea with the modern science of evolution, we may say that the presence of the mind (in the large sense) is one necessary ingredient of living or, in other words, the same particularized will to live which played its part in the gradual formation of the functioning structures must be still present for their continuation, and must not run contrary to the conditions which provided for their formation in the course of their evolution in Nature. Briefly, 'bad thoughts' are unnatural thoughts, but the good thoughts provided for in the meditational reverence in the centres – and helped by various symbols and images – are natural and also conducive to further growth and improvement. In the course of evolution the beneficial habits of structure and function were preserved, and the bad were eliminated.

All this may be condensed down to a statement that the yogis believe in – and tell us that they 'see' and anyhow know – that there is a 'subtle body' (*sūkshma sharīra*), one part of which is especially concerned with the welfare of the dense body. This part (named *prānamayakosha* – vessel or body composed of *prāna*) is in a sense the brain of the body, in that it contains the body-memory which marshals all the newly incoming elements from food and air into their proper places (something like the ring-master in a circus) without which when introduced into the body they would not fall into line and do their parts, for the newly-incoming materials have to respond to the 'obediences' which have been stored in the long process of evolution in Nature in this 'brain of the body'. Think, for example, of the vast number of 'habits' from the past which are coordinated in the course of the development of a child in its mother's womb, all taking place under the direction of this inner mechanism. One is almost tempted to call it automation, or mechanical brain, and would do so but for the fact that it was compounded from the life – or mind – element, which is still there and is still responsive to what is going on.

It will easily be seen that this subtle body (*prānamayakosha*) can have its natural functioning (its governing function) interfered with from two sides – the outside and the inside. Food, clothing, shelter, exercise, rest – all such outside matters, if contrary to the natural 'laws' of the body, will conflict with the built-in power of the 'ring-master' which maintains the body's proper functioning condition. On the other hand, bad thoughts – unnatural thoughts – will also injure it, from the inside. Hence the need for the yogi to take only healthy food and avoid the coarse or stimulating, to wear light clothing, to sit in a healthy posture in a clean place with an adequate temperature, to do some exercise (*āsanas*), etc. Hence the need at the same time for him to think only good thoughts, which are in accord with the five restraints (*yamas*) and the five observances (*niyamas*).[1]

It is significant that when Patanjali takes up the question

1. See Chapter 3.

of how to deal with bad thoughts which may arise during meditation or at other times, he says, as has been quoted before in a different context:

When there is annoyance by bad thoughts, let there be reflection to the contrary. Reflection to the contrary is: The bad thought of injury, etc.[1], whether as done, caused to be done, or approved, whether preceded by greed, anger, or infatuation, whether mild, medium, or strong, results in endless pain and error.[2]

Now, when the mode of bodily living is good and when the thoughts are good, there comes the blessing of abundant vitality. This is real health, and this health is felt *as such*. This health or vitality is *prāna*. The idea is that this is a third something, which is added when there is rightness in both bodily living and mental thinking or picturing. This third something is the divine life in the body, not provided by any of the variety of materials on the one hand, not provided by any of the powers of the mind on the other hand, but welling up (an inadequate expression) in proportion to the harmony of the two.

It will have been noticed that these ideas relate very closely to modern interest in psychosomatic disorders. A very large percentage of hospital cases are of the psychosomatic kind. The science of yoga deals with this situation by pointing out in advance the proneness of the modern human, with his new habits and his new worries and his highly stimulating new sex-theories, which are often mere excuses for unnatural over-indulgence. Next, it points out the value – and incidentally the pleasure – of natural living and good thinking, and some practice of good posture in standing, sitting, walking, or lying down, as an antidote to the under-use (*tamas*) and over-use (*rajas*) of different parts of this precious body of ours. This science should be a ray of hope. It should be a matter of great rejoicing to modern man to find that his diseases are so largely psychosomatic, for now he knows how to avoid them, and no doubt this will some

1. Any thought contrary to the *yamas* and *niyamas*.
2. *Yoga Sūtras*, ii, 33, 34.

day be done by a generation wiser and more natural than ours.

These are matters for the waking life, but also if there is going to be sleep with proper relaxation of the body (allowing for the full functioning of the 'brain of the body'), and proper relaxation of the emotions and mind, preceded by good thoughts, there will be found on awakening a refreshment, rejuvenation, and vitality of physical living which can only be described as a physical divine blessing and even as a veritable participation in the Presence.

This would seem to be the right place in which to include some reflections upon the yogic outlook upon the body in relation to modern knowledge. We will therefore consider how our various limbs and organs arose – a matter with which the yogis, being practical people, do not generally trouble themselves, but which nevertheless is interesting here as bearing on the theory of life.

It is a well-known idea in modern physiological thought that the limbs and organs of the body represent 'lapsed intelligence.' The elementary organism has more function than structure. The amorphous movements of the amoeba, for example, serve various functions such as ingestion, propulsion, and elimination. In the course of evolution organs and limbs are gradually developed so that there are localized structures for the receipt of sensations and the performance of actions. These structures, gradually formed by many repetitions of use, constitute material habit, so that what at first required attention (such as it was) later on became reflex mechanism. Thus the body grew, with its vascular, muscular, and neural systems; after that, bodily operations were performed largely without any conscious knowledge of the established mechanism. Very few people know (or need to know) how their arms and legs work, still less their eyes and ears, still less their breathing, digestion, or circulation of blood.

It is not suggested that the intelligence which formed our limbs and organs was specifically directed to their formation, but that the conscious effort to do certain things brought about these adaptations to the environment. Thus the desire to eat gradually formed a mouth. It was not, however, that a mouth was desired. We must draw a sharp line of demarcation between knowledge and action. The organs which were built under a system of trial and error, backed only by some instinct or desire or impulse to live and to enjoy life, are even now used by most people without knowledge of their mechanism. Even the planning of actions by our advanced intelligence, which has more and more replaced the system of trial and error, knows only the use of the organs, and even today they are being slightly modified, and are especially becoming more sensitive and delicate by use. In the use of the end-organs of the arm, for example, it is noticeable that men generally use the hand (grasping tools) more than the fingers and women use the fingers more than the hand, with corresponding developments and refinements.

In the process of trial and error the will to try again and again with slightly different aims got encouragement by success. It had its limitations, and could be discouraged, but on the whole it had success and survival value. There was no doubt a very elementary amount of reason also, even in the tendency of the organism to try and try again in a slightly different way, as in the case of the paramecium when it backs off after a failure to get food, shifts its angle a little, and tries again, and again.

Then as reason grew, the trial-and-error method grew less and knowledge increased. Memories were formed in the mind; theories built upon them and actions based upon these were more and more successful. So reason developed, which we call 'the higher mind'. This, and all the other structures, while very efficient within very specific functions, are also limitations. Thus our human legs and feet are adapted for walking, but the hind legs of the kangaroo only for jumping. There is disadvantage as well as advantage in having these limbs.

In the light of this fact that the human being does not know how his body works, but that it surely responds to his desires, which is seen in every home when the babe begins to walk but does not know what legs are for until afterwards, it is not surprising that the teachers of yoga in India who instruct their pupils in various exercises simply tell them what to do and let them find the results by experience. It is the natural method. In consequence of this, when we read the statements of the classical books on *hatha-yoga*, we find a great indefiniteness and a certain amount of confusion and difference of opinion as to what actually happens *in the body* when the exercises are done, but no confusion or difference as to the results.

We have come to the point in evolution at which our thinking of the body has some effect upon it. Definite concentration upon (or in) an organ of the body does stimulate it. Thus, when it is said, for example, that a definite force resides latent or almost latent at a centre near the base of the spine, and concentration of attention on (or better in) that place stimulates it into activity, it is understood that something will be aroused, but that when aroused it will in the main follow its own bent and produce its own effects.

In this connexion the standard knowledge which we have considered in our two previous chapters about 'the serpent power' (Kundalinī), the vital airs (*vāyus* and *prānas*), the channels (*nādis*) in which these travel, and other such matters is seen to be reasonable.

In the old psychology of India this thinking, planning mind (*manas*) of ours was regarded only as an adjunct of 'the ten organs' (five of sense and five of action). It grew up in service to them. All the contents (pictures or ideas) in that mind are brought into it by the senses. The objects of the world are reflected into it, and the impressions thus received, as in a camera, are retained and stored, and can be thrown on the screen of memory by an act of will similar to that which occurs when hands or legs are used for definite actions.

So much is this mind a development for the convenience of the body that it came to be called the eleventh organ (*indriya*). By means of it there can be comparison of what is now seen with what has been seen before, which is 'recognition' and, later, the recalling of things on the screen of imagination by 'memory'. There can be quietness or inaction of the mind, as of the bodily organs. It can be called into action in specific ways, just as the limbs can, though it is much more 'amoebic' than the body is.

When, however, there has been long and definite training or use of the mind in special subjects there is here too a tendency to 'structure', resulting in beliefs and prejudices or, in general, inclinations and, very often, decision by precedent, with its tendency to 'lapsed intelligence' even in the mind. And so, just as we need a variety of exercises (especially of breathing and posturing, as prescribed in yoga) for the body, so we also need meditation (*dhyāna*) for the mind, *not* for the purpose of establishing mental habits or 'conditioning the mind', but for the purpose of keeping the whole machinery supple and available for use when required. Such meditation, as explained in our Chapter 4, begins with the selection of a subject of thought, called a ground (*bhūmi*), and then proceeds to reflect upon that subject until every possible thought in reference to it has been brought forward and considered. In physical exercises (to make the comparison of mental and physical) at a given time the ground (or *bhūmi*) may be, for example, the neck, the eyes, the spine, the lungs, and in a given exercise we proceed to activate all the functions of the 'ground', some of which may otherwise be subject to neglect, especially in our rather sedentary or otherwise specialized modern life.

Behind these organs are the senses proper, or rather sensations. We experience sounds, feelings, colours, savours, and odours. These are even more 'within' than the sense organs. These 'experiences in consciousness' are *varieties* of knowing or 'something measured off' (*tanmātras*) from or in the totality of our consciousness or environment. There is something very difficult to understand about these varieties of knowing, for they do not partake of the character of the objects seen, but are in the nature of awakenings in consciousness which occur in the presence of certain things.

So deep indeed, so 'inner' are these *tanmātras* or things measured off in our consciousness that several scriptures speak of our organs as only serving them. The divine being is then spoken of as hearing without ears, seeing without eyes, etc. This is a case in which we must accept 'what is'. The theory of Indian philosophy or psychology in the matter is that each man will sooner or later reach that spiritual or divine position, and will then hear without ears, etc., our present living method being only a schooling for that, in which we develop the 'powers' of our consciousness, or our innate potentialities.

In this schooling we attend to one thing after another, as in an ordinary school. The children in a class may have arithmetic at 9 o'clock, history at 10 o'clock, and literature at 11 o'clock, and they must drop the 9 o'clock thoughts and memories about arithmetic during the 10 o'clock history period, in which period the arithmetic knowledge has become 'lapsed intelligence' in the subconsciousness of the lower mind, though the *thinking ability* gained by doing arithmetic is partly active in that history period. Yet there is also to some extent 'lapsed intelligence' even in the higher mind, as predisposing that thinking mind to facility in the specific functioning peculiar or particular to arithmetic.

These *tanmātras* or basic sensations can be regarded as divided or separated in a manner analogous to a spectrum, leading us to agree to the proposition that ultimately they will merge into the one white light of pure consciousness, such oneness not implying any loss but only a complete lack of separateness. This implies an inner completion or completeness in and at the back of the mind.

It is notable that in dreams our visions are 'more real' than those we can make by deliberate visualization. Try to visualize a rose and you may feel it to be a poor similitude, but dream the same rose and it will be as good, clear, and strong as if it were seen. Or, in the hypnotic state, when there is the suggestion of a rose, the vision will have all the qualities of the real article for sight, touch, and smell. The theory is thus tenable that the mental residues in the 'subconscious' are as good in sense-qualities as the sense-experience ever was. There is no fading there.

We may also recognize that fundamentally our seeing, hearing, etc., are even now beyond the organs of sight, etc.

Coming now to the 'vitality' (*prāna*), we recognize that there is something in the body that gives *quality* to sensations and to our actions. Two things are involved in this. One is the aliveness of the sense-organs. The other is the attentiveness of the consciousness. Both are improving by the schooling method of 'one thing at a time', and thus there is an added 'vitality' of living when they are in harmony.

THE USE OF SOUNDS IN YOGA PRACTICE

In India one often meets with the use of incantations – repetitions of words regarded as having an effect. Sometimes this is thought of as an effect upon the mind, as in the very common case where a person who is worried or in trouble mutters the word '*Rām*' over and over again to himself. The word 'incantation' is perhaps too dramatic to describe this simple repetition; it conjures up rather a picture of the witches in *Macbeth*. It does come within the definition, however, because the name *Rām* is generally felt to have some bodily and mental effect, in addition to its conventional meaning.

In the far distant past, Rāma was a king in India. Some have called him the ideal king on account of his valour and goodness and wisdom, and he is listed as a veritable Incarnation (*avatāra*) of Vishnu, the preserver of all life.

The troubled person in this case has probably heard the story of Tulsi Das's abridged *Rāmāyana*, or the life of Rāma, over and over again as a child at his mother's knee, so this particular *japa* (repetition or muttering) has for him the comfort of the childhood background, the thought that somehow Rāma will even now, from his empyrean or from his mystic presence, send some help, and, thirdly, the feeling that the very word thus repeated soothes both body and mind.

This *japa* could not strictly be called an incantation however. It is altogether too passive. The yogi is a very positive person, and though his *mantras* are nearly always addressed to a form of deity, and though they are often couched in terms of a relation to that deity from which he expects to benefit, his conception is clearly that of one who is doing something requiring an effort which is calculated to produce an effect.

It may be that the name of a divinity will help him to keep his mind on a conception and keep other thoughts away while he passes from meditation into *samādhi*, a *samādhi* (contemplation) in which he absorbs the qualities of that divinity.

In these circumstances it would not be very profitable for him to enter upon the *samādhi* without a fairly clear conception of what the divinity stands for. This it may be assumed the Hindu yogi already has, though it will be improved in his meditation by his thinking and in his *samādhi* by his intuitions respecting it.

I am assuming now that while using the name or the formula of a divinity the devotee is doing only what is called *samprajnāta samādhi*, that is, he has a definite object in mind. To understand this position it will be well at this point to digress a little and review the significance of this kind of *samādhi*. For this we may again refer to Patanjali.

The contemplation (*samādhi*) proposed by that most authoritative exponent of yoga, can be firstly of a kind called cognitive (*samprajnāta*), when it is accompanied by (1) inspection or discernment (*vitarka*) of an object, (2) investigation or consideration (*vichāra*) of the class, attributes, and value of the object, including those roots of classification, the subtle 'senses' (*tanmātras*), (3) delight (*ānanda*), or (4) a sense of one's own power or attainment (*asmitā*), which, literally, means 'I-am-ness'.

Secondly, it can be of a kind called non-cognitive (*asamprajnāta*). This occurs when the contemplation is without any motive of knowing, understanding, enjoying the presence of an object or the thought of it, or any thrill of personal satisfaction, which conceals a deep egotism. It is, as it were, an attempt to reach into the region beyond mind, with no worldly desire of any kind whatsoever. Such a motive may come about from faith (*shraddhā*) in whatever glimpse, mental or otherwise, one may have had into the 'beyond', but will need to be assisted by the vigour and the memory of the vision and the ability to contemplate, and the understanding derived from the practice of the foregoing (*samprajnāta*) method.

Failing this insight and faith, it may be led up to by what Patanjali calls attentiveness to God (*īshwara-pranidhāna*). Some translators have taken the meaning of the word *pranidhāna* to be positive prostration, and the etymology of it does not preclude that as one of its meanings also; there is no objection to it if we understand that we are undertaking something in the mind and, what is more, that highest operation of the mind which is *samādhi*. In this case, indeed, it is implied that whether one has glimpsed the conception of God in an intuition or one has only read or heard about it, one has become completely devoted and attentive to it in all circumstances, as far as one can. In its perfection it would mean an insight into what Jesus was speaking of when he said that five sparrows are sold for two farthings, and yet 'not one of them falls to the ground without my Father'. Such an insight means that the yogic candidate strives to be aware of that absolute Presence.

The foregoing remarks are intended as an introduction to the group of aphorisms or theorems in the *Yoga Sūtras* which constitutes the only reference to God in this *rāja-yoga* manual. They are provided for in *Sūtras*, i, 16–23, immediately after which we have the following:

'God is the perfect spirit (*purusha-vishesha*) not affected by containers (bodies) of troubles (*kleshas*), actions (*karmas*), or their results (*vipākas*).'[1]

This means that he is different from ordinary men. Although these at their root – the real men – are also unaffected, in the world they let themselves be affected, through their ignorance of their own true nature, which yoga seeks to alleviate. All things, whether of body or mind, are dependent upon other things, but God is independent, self-existing, and self-originating. So will a man find himself to be, when he achieves the goal of this yoga, which is independence (*kaivalya*). Even now it is so, but it is

1. *Yoga Sūtras*, i, 24. See also Chapter 2 above, with reference to our translation, 'the perfect spirit'.

concealed from his lazy and fearful eyes. The fact is that everyone makes his own decisions, for if we follow another it is because we have chosen to do so, and if we obey a whip it is because we have chosen to obey rather than to suffer. Therefore it is that in the system of *rāja-yoga*, the yogi is attentive to God as the model of what he himself can be or is going to be. The sources of trouble are ignorance, egotism, desire, aversion, and possessiveness.[1]

In Him is the unexcelled source of all knowing.
He was the teacher (*guru*) also of the ancients, being unlimited by time.[2]

In this is concealed, and revealed, the doctrine of food, which is also the doctrine of grace. We have food for the body, for the mind, and for the spirit – the last being 'the bread that cometh down from heaven'. Our own work in all this is only to take what is spread out for us in the field of Nature and of thought – the scientists and the philosophers do not create the truths they discover and expound – and by the Divine.

And now we come to the most important word of power (*mantra*) in all the Hindu scriptures:

His announcer (*vāchaka*) is the sacred word (*pranava*).[3]
Vāchaka is 'stater' rather than mere word. *Pranava* means the word or rather announcement *Om*, which is written ॐ or ॐ
There should be repetition (*japa*) of it, with concentrated thought upon its meaning.[4]

A thorough understanding of this *mantra* will enable the reader or student to understand the nature of all the other *mantras*.

First, it must be clearly stated that the *mantras* used in yoga (many yogis do not use them) are for the purpose of proceeding towards the infinite, not for material gain. They are directed towards Shiva the destroyer, not towards Brahmā the creator. Really, all religion is devotion to either Vishnu or Shiva – to Vishnu as the preserver of life

1. *ibid.*, ii, 3.   2. *ibid.*, i, 25, 26.   3. *ibid.*, i, 27.   4. *ibid.*, i, 28.

or to Shiva as its fulfilment in something beyond. In all India there is only one temple dedicated to Brahmā – at Bhuvaneshwar – and in that temple there is no worship, since Brahmā is, so to say, that aspect of deity which provides for the materiality of the material world.

Hence it must be understood that these *mantras* are intended to help in the achievement of spiritual aims. Therefore *Om* is recited for upward-going, and that is why its three parts, which are the letters a, u, and m, are respectively representatives of body, soul, and spirit. The sound begins with a – the first letter of the alphabet, having utterance of the back of the mouth. It continues with u (short oo) made in the middle of the mouth. It ends with the last of the letters that can be made by the mouth, namely m, by closing the lips at the front end of the series. Therefore, it is argued, when these letters are produced in a continuous glide there is an epitome of all the vocal sounds. And that is why this word is considered to be the announcer of God.

In sounding the word, the a and the u become blended into o, in accordance with Sanskrit phonetics, and so it becomes sounded and written as *Om*.

The m is not an ordinary consonant m sounded with the usual opening of the lips, but is sounded with the lips closed, thus giving a humming sound, especially if prolonged. This is often written with not merely a dot but also a small crescent (lying on the flat of its back) beneath the dot. The crescent represents the continuing sound, for it is always prolonged to some extent – not terminated within the limit of one syllable of time, as it is when it is used in ordinary words. This prolongation is called the *nāda* (sound). Then, after that, we have the dot, called *bindu*, which word ordinarily means a drop, or a globule, or a dot or a point. Here it indicates that the sound terminates in a point in the strictest sense of the word – the sound is not cut off, but dies away in an invisible and undetectable point.

Therefore it is said that the *Om* consists of five things – a, u, and m, *nāda* and *bindu*, the first three being within the field of material speech, the last two indicating a condition beyond it to which the yogi or worshipper aspires. The sacred syllable may be sounded loudly or softly or even silently (that is, mentally), softly being better than loudly, and silently better than softly, since one is aiming within or above. Although, of the three letters, Shiva is represented by the m, he is seated in the *bindu*.

Om is used at the beginning of all spiritual undertakings. The *Bhagavad Gītā* gives us a clear and authentic statement of this in its seventeenth discourse:

'*Om Tat Sat.*' This has been taught as the triple designation of Brahman. With this the Brāhmanas, the Vedas, and the Yajnas were ordained, in the old time.

Therefore, after pronouncing '*Om*', the acts of sacrifice, gift, and austerity done by the students of Brahman are always begun, as stated in the rules.

With '*Tat*', and the rejection of any fruit, acts of sacrifice and austerity, and acts of giving of various kinds are done by those desirous of liberation.

In reference to reality and in reference to goodness the '*Sat*' is used. Similarly, in the case of an act of consecration the word '*Sat*' is used. Steadiness in sacrifice, in austerity, and in giving is also called '*Sat*' and (other) action done for the sake of that is also denominated '*Sat*'.[1]

The purpose of all this explanation is to show something of the meaning involved in what is universally acknowledged in India to be the greatest of all the *mantras*, namely *Om*.

In connexion with this, we may also consider the four levels of every mantric word:

(1) The sound of it;
(2) The meaning of the word;
(3) The idea it embodies;
(4) The spirit (*para*) of it.

In the case of *Om*, these would be: (1) the sound, in which by the prolongation (*nāda*) and the ending in a point (*bindu*) there is a material representation of the entire implication of it; (2) the statement it makes – in this case, the divine

1. Wood, Ernest (trans.), *Bhagavad Gītā Explained*, xvii, 23–7.

presence – which provides a ground of concentration; (3) all the ideas in it – providing ground of meditation; and (4) the root of it, or the spiritual meaning – the 'colour' of it in the spectrum of the one sound, regarded as an axis of creation and therefore as a 'Jacob's ladder' into the 'heaven'.

Mantras cannot be made by everybody. They have to be provided through or by a competent seer (*mantrakāra*). In the case of *Om*, the source of it is regarded as nothing less than the triple divinity; it came to man as a revelation, not as a construct of his own. It is therefore potent in all four respects.

Now, as to the sounding – there is option as to length, and the yogi must generally use his own feeling and intuition about this. But it must be used as one syllable only. And generally the m sound will be at least twice as long as the o sound, which should be full and round, as in the word home.

In the ending of it the ideal pronunciation would taper it off to an imperceptible point. Every written or drawn line ends in a line, not in a point; in other words, it is abrupt. The sound should not end abruptly like that. This is possible with sound, and the tapering does not involve any particular or great length. It is in the power of the reciter to make it short or long. On an ordinary occasion the o may well last about two seconds and the m about four seconds. The *Dhyānaḥindu Upanishad* says that the sounding of the m should be as uninterrupted as a flow of oil, and as long as the sound of a bell.

There should also be thought or intentness upon its meaning. This will cause the exclusion of other thoughts. There should be a grasp of the fullness of the meaning, fed and increased by prior meditations. And in the ending of it there would be, in its perfection, an experience of its spiritual root.

The three parts of *Om* are allotted to the three great Gods (*devas*) of the one divine Being. The a represents Brahmā, the creator; the u Vishnu, the preserver; and the m Shiva, the destroyer. Brahmā and Vishnu work together. Other *mantras* are limited, but this *Om* is all-inclusive, and so it represents God (Brahman) in his fullness.[1]

In order to observe the amount of thought or material for meditation packed into this *mantra* – for it is so important that no part of its meaning should be neglected – let us consider the significance of the three deities.

The relation between Brahmā – that aspect or function of deity to whom was assigned the work of creation – and Vishnu, the preserver, is well indicated in a story which relates that after Brahmā had created the world, which he did by meditation on the word (*vāch*) and sound, he looked at his creation and was not pleased, because it was 'dead and motionless'. Then he prayed for life for it, which he could not provide. In response to this, Vishnu entered into that dead world and filled it with life.

Another of the many stories in the books of ancient legends (*Purānas*) is still clearer. It begins by relating that the great *deva* Nārāyana, Vishnu, the soul and life of the Universe, thousand-eyed and omniscient, was reclining upon his couch, which was the body of the great serpent *Sesha* or *Ananta* (endless time) which lay coiled up on the waters of space, as it was the night of being.[2] Then in the story, Brahmā, the great creator of the world of being, called *Sat*, came to him and touched him with his hand, and asked, 'Who art thou?' This resulted in an argument between them as to who was the greater. Suddenly there arose before them a huge pillar of fire and light, incomparable and indescribable, which astonished the disputants so much

1. It is to be remembered that Brahman or Brahma means the entire godhead or deity, the source of the three deities which are functional towards a world, and Brahmā (with the long a at the end) is one of the three functional deities. An interesting resemblance to this is the way in which we sort ourselves out mentally when we wake up – we notice the objective things and say to ourselves, 'Here we are again', then we remember who we are, and then we begin to plan the purpose of the day.

2. This means that the world was in a dissolved or latent condition (*pralaya*); the old cosmogony of India provides for alternate long periods of manifestation and latency.

that they forgot their quarrel and agreed to search for the end of so wonderful a thing.

Vishnu plunged downwards for a thousand years, but he could not find its base, and Brahmā flew upwards for a thousand years, but he could not find its top, so both returned baffled. Then the pillar opened, and Shiva, whose nature is joy (*ānanda*), stood before them and, having demonstrated his superiority by means of the pillar of light, explained that he and they were three functions of one supreme being, of which he, Shiva, was the chief, and that in the coming age they would work together in the business of a new world until, the undertaking being finished, they would both be with their overlord again.

In this trinity or triple form (*trimūrti*) Shiva, it will be remembered, is called the destroyer, the form of deity who winds up the affairs of a world or of a man. Into Shiva or that background (for he also is a function) both the material side and the life side of things will be dissolved. The school, so to say, will be wound up, some of the scholars having learned everything, and others being laid off for a rest, pending the opening of another school.

The function of the destroyer has to be carefully understood, because Shiva is the patron of yogis, who are bringing their 'schooling' to an end. It means that Shiva operates what in the human mind would be called the *purpose* of the undertaking called manifestation. When that work is finished and the living beings have got out of it all they need for their spiritual awakening and self-realization the manifestation is dissolved. As well as the simile of a school one may use that of dolls. When a doll has done its work it must be destroyed or put away.

It might be better to call the three great gods *custodians* of (1) the material, (2) the living minds, and (3) the spiritual purpose, rather than simply the creator, preserver, and destroyer. These last three terms are too intent upon the material side of things. In India every *mantra* is addressed to one or other of the three great gods, or to the god's wife or consort, and the words or letters pronounced are in some direct or indirect way connected with them, and therefore with their functions and powers. In this way both the meaning and the very sound of the word are taken to have a specific potency. It is to be noticed that in everything we do we need something material or static, plus something of mind-function, and something of an ultimate purpose – however remote the last may seem, it being nevertheless present throughout. Even the modern physicist cannot manage entirely without corpuscularity.

It has already been remarked that in ordinary affairs we walk in order to stop walking (having 'got there'), and we think in order to stop thinking (having solved the problem). So also we live in order to stop living; the schooling is finished and Vishnu hands us over to Shiva, so to speak.

Although not strictly a *mantra* of yoga, but rather a prayer used for centuries by men of the highest caste, and now by anybody having the right understanding and intention, the *mantra* termed the *Gāyatrī* should be included in this book. It is:

Om. Bhūr bhuvah swah: Tat savitur varenyam bhargo devasya dhīmahi; Dhiyo yo nah prachodayāt. Om.

For this I give the following translation in my *Yoga Dictionary*:

We meditate on the most excellent glory of that divine Sun (or Source); may That direct our understanding.

The divine Sun (or Source) here is to be understood as 'That'. with the significance imparted to it by a capital 'T'. This word 'That' is often used in *Upanishads* and other scriptural works to indicate the Beyond, while there is another pronoun, *idam* (this), which indicates all the expanded world of matter and mind.

The use of we and our in the *mantra*, one may remark in passing, is very pleasing. Thus, even when, as is usual, the devotee is reciting this alone, he is thinking of others, not only of himself.

In the concluding portion, 'May That direct our understanding', the word 'direct' is not quite meaningful enough.

To bring out the meaning of the word fully we need to use the two words 'direct' and 'impel' – perhaps 'inspire' would be the best. It indicates that the divine effulgence is what we have called the Original Power, as the divine (in *devasya*) means that. The word 'power' is more than scientific, since in science power acts upon something and expends itself, but this is ineffable and inexpendable, being creator, supporter, and withdrawer all in one. Wherever there is enlightening, there is the presence of all three – the coming of something new, the sustaining of it, and the withdrawal of old wrong or imperfect view. That original power is always present in all our being and qualities and actions as has been shown, as, for example, when we find and have confidence in the 'floating in walking'.[1] Such a discovery is a partial liberation.

That such a *mantra* should be used as the morning prayer – at daybreak, in olden times – indicates that the devotee wishes to remember, in all his work of the day, that the purpose behind it all was the reaching of That. Similarly, as already mentioned, when the 'students of Brahman' recite the *Om Tat Sat* at the beginning of an undertaking they remind themselves that though they have an object in view by their undertaking in the world, it is not really their aim, but only something directly or indirectly leading (and by them intended to lead) to the goal referred to by That (*Tat*). That is the Reality (*Sat*) which they affirm.

With the *Om* the devotee thus reminds himself that all this is being done also in the Presence of the high trinity. At the same time by pronouncing the word he is being an agent of that Presence in the region of human speech. The *mantra* is (in every case) the Deity within that limitation. Just as every hand is a presence of 'hand', when it is united with arm and body, but if such things or shapes had been merely lying about on the floor they would not have been hands, so also everything is what it is because of its union with that Presence.

Bhūr, bhuvah, and *swah* remind the worshipper that this is

1. See the discussion of Original Power in Chapter 2.

taking place in three worlds at once. These worlds are often spoken of as *lokas*, e.g. *bhuvar-loka*, the terminal h having given place to r for the sake of euphony. *Loka* means an inhabited world. The three worlds, are usually taken to mean the world, an intermediate world, and heaven, but some have given them a wider significance, while others have added four more and thus refer to seven worlds or planes of being.

Others again consider that the three refer respectively to our physical, emotional, and mental states. Those are to be regarded very objectively, as the person in the form of mind and thoughts can exist apart from the body, as 'subtle body'. Thus the three regions are not merely vibratory levels, but are populated habitats, and the *swah* or *swarga* is described in the *Purānas* as a kingdom in which meritorious people, who are not in the grip of passions or bad emotions, enjoy long periods of great happiness in the interval between death and birth.[1] It is considered that the thoughts of living persons reach into that state only when they are good, as it is a region or rather state well guarded and too fine (*sūkshma*) for anything low or ugly or sad to enter. This does not exclude beautiful trees, mountains, rivers, horses, elephants, and people, but does exclude roughness, ugliness, quarrel, disease, dust, excessive heat, cold, etc.

Some others, again, associate the three (*bhūh*, etc.) with the first three *chakras*, counting from below, and this agrees with the idea that these three are especially concerned with the objective, material affairs, threefold as material, emotional and represented in mind – the field of attachment to things. The recital of the three indicates the desire to bring all three within the scope of the prayer. Very often after the *Om* at the end of such a prayer, the word *shāntih* is recited three times. It means 'peace'.

Three states are also mentioned in another way in Hindu philosophy – the familiar Waking, Dreaming, and Sleeping series. In dreaming there is no mental control, but a flow of

1. See e.g. *the Garuda Purāna*, xiv, trans. Ernest Wood.

pictures following the line of least resistance emotionally and mentally. These dreams are emotionally healing, provided they are not analysed, but are simply received and allowed to carry their own lessons, which can be well known intuitively on waking if they are so dwelt upon without direction or desire for a little while. The third state, deep, dreamless sleep, is not really unconscious, but is beyond the picturing and emotional flow. One wakes from it with great refreshment and encouragement, and the memory, 'I slept well; I enjoyed that sleep', which is quite different from an inference that I feel well now and so must have slept well. A fourth (*turīya*) state is that reached in deep *samādhi*.

In general, it is held that all movements produce sound, though much of it is not heard by us on account of the limitation of our ears. The kind of sound depends upon the nature of the object and of its movement. And since things are not merely things, but have specific qualities and actions (according to circumstances, of course) as part of their being, the sounds produced are specific to those producers. Further, since mental desire (which involves a picture, however vague) precedes every form (whether produced individually as in the case of a man or with accidental collectiveness, as in the case of a rainstorm) the sound produced is its natural name. A competent *mantrakāra* (*mantra* composer) could make a *mantra* having an affinity with an archetype,[1] or expressing an idea, or representing one of

1. An 'archetype' is the fullest expression possible for an 'axis of creation' in a given *loka*. Thus, for example, a triangle on paper, in two dimensions, is the maximum expression of a structural principle. It could not be more perfect. It has reached perfection. If the same principle were in a three-dimensional locus the perfect expression would be a tetrahedron. It has reached perfection. So there can be such a thing as a perfect man, or, for that matter, a perfect house, or a perfect pen. The 'axes of creation' meet the environment or come into a locus.

Apply the idea to colours and you can think of perfect red, for example. Or to sounds. Thus all things are the result of the interplay of the axes of creation, which in the material world is primarily sound, since word expresses idea. Hence the 'word' which was with God in the beginning and indeed was God (not merely a separate agent) is the perfect man,

those spiritual principles (or axes of creation) which may be considered to be responsible for the fact that our world is not a mere heap of disconnected and characterless things, but has perfect classification wherever we may look – among men or animals or plants or things.

So – to go back to the very root – Shiva is concerned with the will, the purpose and fulfilment of life, Vishnu with the wisdom which is the knowing of the value of things for the life which is doing its living, and Brahmā with the thoughts which lead to material form.

These three functions are also related to will (*ichchhā*), wisdom (*jnāna*), and activity (*kriyā*). In this connexion it has to be remembered that thought is the activity of the mind, and in all these three we are talking of some divine functions beyond mind, which, however, express themselves in our minds as will, wisdom, and thought leading to activity. Therefore it is that a *mantra* is regarded as a 'sound-body' for a specific function of the divine 'movement' called a deva[1] – divine being or god.

The sounding of the *mantra* correctly forms, then, a definite impulse from its proper principal and principle. We all know that music, and even particular notes of the scale, affect various parts of our bodies. I once knew a man from the remote interior of Africa who maintained and demonstrated that by the rhythms and sounds of his drums, learned from an old master of the art in the depths of Africa, he could cause the shoulders and other parts of the bodies of his hearers to move involuntarily, in various ways, as, for example, the legs to dance. In some sense we could say, therefore, that correct *mantras* would constitute a sort of telepathy reaching not merely from mind to mind but from mind through sound to the affecting of bodies and even things.

As the Brahmins retained the *Gāyatrī* exclusively for them-

the archetype of man. If man were to go beyond that he would cease to be man, and burst forth from this cocoon (as it were) into something else, having 'gone to the Father'.

1. Not to be confused with a so-called 'deva evolution' – a misuse of the word.

selves (presumably originally on the theory that they alone were qualified to understand it) the Tāntric leaders provided another sacred verse, called *Brahma-gāyatrī*, for the use of others. This runs:

Parameshwarāya vidmahe paratattwāya dhīmahi.

We are understandingly awake to the Supreme God; we meditate upon the Supreme Truth.

Tan no Brahma prachodayāt.

May that Brahman direct us.[1]

Another *mantra* in much use is '*Om namo Nārāyanāya*'. The literal meaning is '*Om*, a bow to the supreme spirit.' It is called the eight-syllabled *mantra* of the supreme being, Nārāyana. Nārāyana is the divine and universal Self, and is also described as the Son of Man, perfect man, what man will be when perfect. More fully translated, our *mantra* is 'In the presence of the divine, devotion to the primal man' – or perfect man or archetypal man. It is as though a Christian devotee were to distinguish very closely or lucidly the distinction between Jesus as Son of God and Jesus as Son of Man. In the former capacity he declared himself the same as the rest of us – 'Ye are all sons of God' – but in the latter capacity he showed himself on the several occasions when the term was used, to be perfect man – what men will be when by their endeavours (and especially the endeavours to fulfil the two commandments to love God and man) they have given full birth to themselves and achieved the fruition or full growth which is the object of their sojourn in this world.

Nara means man; *ayana*, the coming – already, however, come in the model of the Incarnation, the *Avatāra*. In this view, every man has sooner or later to give birth to his own perfection – in which sense the struggling being of today is the father of his own future perfect self, or perfect man.

To make the most of every detail of a *mantra* the ancients gave a meaning to every syllable. In this case, says Yajnavalkya, 'Through *Om* Brahma is presented; through *na*, Vish-

1. From the *Mahānirvāna Tantra*, iii, 109–11, given in Arthur Avalon's *Garland of Letters*.

nu; through *mo*, Rudra (Shiva); through *na*, Īshwara; through *rā*, the spread-out universe; through *ya*, the real man (the *purusha*); through *nā*, the Incarnation; and through *ya*, the supreme self (*paramātmā*).' It comes as a surprise when one first sees the amount of combined cosmogony and theogony which is packed into one composite idea expressed in a small *mantra*. Meditation for long periods becomes possible in the building of the *mantra* in the mind of the devotee, and very great contemplation (*samādhi*) becomes possible in its completed use.

In the *mantra*, *namo* is really *namah*, which means that one bows, hailing with a wise joy that is receptive, not splurging, the God, combining power and virtue, that is named Nārāyana. The *namah* has become *namo* to satisfy a rule of euphony which blends the ending of the word with the soft letter which begins the next – one of those dozen or so rules which make the Sanskrit diction flow so smoothly and suit it to the making of *mantras* and of speech which is, so to speak, healing at the same time that it is informative.

It is significant that the eight-syllabled '*Om namo Nārā-yanāya*' is called the *Tārasāra Mantra*, the essential way of crossing, as *tāra* means 'crossing over this mundane existence', and *sāra* means 'extracted essence'. It is fully described in the *Tārasārā Upanishad*. In that there is a wealth of theistic imagery associated with each syllable, as also in the *Nārāyana Upanishad*.

It is related in the *Tārasāra Upanishad* that one Bharadwaja approached the great sage, Yajnavalkya, and asked him what is the means to cross over this worldly existence and be done with it as such, and he replied that the means of crossing (the *tāraka*) is '*Om Namo Nārāyanāya*'. *Om* we have already considered. It is of the nature of the true Self, which every person can find if he really looks into the depths of himself to see what it is that is himself, with a seeing that is himself seeing himself, and not seeing merely his works. The artist must look at himself, not merely at the pictures which he has painted. This is a kind of double looking, which is conscious, for example, of the foot pressing the ground while the ground resists the free movement of the foot. To become 'foot-conscious' to our very roots is the real aim of experience.

The idea of 'crossing over' can be conveyed by thinking of life (that is, the long series of lives) as a journey. One old writer remarked, however, that there is no travelling on this road. The journey is really the progressive awakening of consciousness. This involves becoming implicated in things in the earlier stages and afterwards becoming released from them.

Even the small matter of paying attention to something is a 'descent into hell', a self-restriction by the acceptance of a limitation. It is thus that concentration limits or binds. This life becomes 'one thing after another' instead of 'all at once'. Thus time arises, because actions are one after another. Then time becomes external for us, because all beings are holding on to things and moving (or changing) only with reluctance and slowness.[1] Then we find ourselves accepting external time. As mind has produced forms it has also produced time, and we find ourselves in the midst of both as long as we pay attention or concentrate on anything. Later on as part of the awakening we become interested in mind, and later still in the pure consciousness in which there is no time.

In the course of the external time-sequence which represents the mass-movement of the whole boat-load of beings who constitute our world there are thus stages or eras. The present era is considered the worst, and is called the 'black age'. It is regarded as the age in which the human race is most involved in material things, and therefore is in great bondage. If, however, one can in the midst of all this clamour give attention to the spirit 'within' oneself and

1. First there is *āvarana* (limitation, restriction, exclusion, partial covering-up), and then *vikshepa* (action, creation). Then the devotion to external continuity of things which is in our character (though we may not call it devotion but merely desire) associates the doing or creation with the inert or *tāmasic* power (of Brahmā), and then one has 'material time', or external time. Ultimately time will not stop, but will dissolve. It is only the actions of the beings (all beings; including what we call minerals), while the material being of these beings constitutes extensity (giving rise to the illusion of space).

'above' all this, one is acquiring more intelligence and will-power, that is, awakening, than one would be likely to do in easier circumstances.

Very much allied in character to the *Nārāyana Mantra* is the '*mantra* of the sixteen names', which comes to us from the *Kalisantārana Upanishad*, and is said to be especially useful in overcoming the distracting conditions of our present 'dark age' (*kali yuga*). These names help the yogi to keep common outward thoughts from occupying his attention, while the mind does its inward-going. The *mantra* has not sixteen different names, as might be expected, but three names, all indicating Vishnu, arranged as follows:

Hare, Rāma; Hare, Rāma; Rāma, Rāma; Hare, Hare; Hare, Krishna; Hare, Krishna; Krishna, Krishna; Hare, Hare.[1]

Another such personal *mantra* is the five-divisioned, eighteen-syllabled *mantra* to Shrī Krishna, addressed to him especially in his boy form, when he was growing up among the cow-keeping people of Brindāvan. This *mantra* was given to me, with his very strong recommendations, nearly fifty years ago by Sir S. Subrahmanya Iyer, Chief Justice of the Madras High Court, who in private life was devoted to yoga. He told me that its value had first been impressed upon him earlier by one whom he regarded as a great occultist, T. Subba Rao.

I give it now with some explanations which I translated at the time from the *Gopālatāpani* and *Krishna Upanishads*.

The *mantra* runs:

> Klīm Krishnāya –
> Govindāya –
> Gopī-jana –
> Vallabhāya –
> Swāhā.[2]

1. *Hare* is pronounced as two syllables, ha and re. E is sounded as in the word 'grey' and is always the same in all Sanskrit words. The a in Hare is short, like the a in 'America' or 'India'. In Rāma the a is like a in 'father', so that the whole word rhymes with 'farmer'.

2. For correct pronunciation: ī as ee; ā as in 'father'; a as in 'India'; o as in 'home'; i as in 'India'.

The following, which is a very close translation, gives some idea of the wealth of imagery connected with the deities and their symbols.

Once the Sages came to the great Brahmā and asked: Who is the Supreme God? Whom does Death fear? Through the knowledge of what does all become known? What makes this world continue on its course?

He replied: Shrī Krishna verily is the Supreme God. Death is afraid of Govind (Shrī Krishna). By knowing the Lord of Gopī-jana (Shrī Krishna) the whole world is known. By Swāhā the world goes on evolving.

Then they questioned him again: Who is Krishna? Who is Govinda? Who is the Lord of Gopī-jana? What is Swāhā?

He replied: 'Krishna is he who destroys all wrong, who is the knower of all things, who, on earth, is known through the great teaching. The Lord of Gopī-jana is he who guides all conditioned beings. Swāhā is his power. He who meditates on these, repeats the *mantra*, worships him, becomes immortal.

Again they asked him: What is his form? What is his *mantra*? What is his worship?'

He replied: He who has the form of a protector of cows (the verses of the great teaching). The cloud-coloured youth (the colour of the fathomless deep). He who sits at the root of the tree (whose spreading branches are the creation and evolution of the ages). He whose eyes are like the full-blown lotus (always resting in the pure lotus hearts of his devotees). He whose raiment is of the splendour of lightning (shining by its own light). He who is two-armed (the life and the form). He who is possessed of the sign of wisdom with which the silent sages are initiated. He who wears a garland of flowers (the string of globes or planets). He who is seated on the centre of the golden lotus (at the heart of all). Who meditates upon him becomes free.

His is the *mantra* of five parts. The first is Klīm Krishnāya. Klīm is the seed of attraction. The second is Govindāya. The third is Gopī-jana. The fourth is Vallabhāya. The fifth and last is Swāhā.

Klīm – to Krishna – to the Giver of Knowledge – to the Lord of the Cowherds – Swāhā.

Om. Adoration to the Universal Form, the Source of all Protection, the Goal of Life, the Ruler of the Universe, and the Universe itself.

Om. Adoration to the Embodiment of Wisdom, the Supreme

Delight, Krishna, the Lord of Cowherds! To the Giver of Knowledge, adoration!

Sir John Woodroffe refers to *Klīm*, a meaningless word with which this *mantra* begins, in other connexions in his book, *The Garland of Letters*.[1] He calls it the *Kāmabīja*, *kāma* meaning love. This word *kāma* – though much maligned because of its inferior associations – is positively divine when in accordance with duty and not an impulse of passion. Referring to the general principle, Shrī Krishna, as a divine Incarnation (*avatāra*), indeed the fullest Incarnation (*pūrnāvatāra*) according to the Hindus, advises his disciple Arjuna to act in life only 'with a view to the welfare of the world (people)'.

He further explains his own position as Incarnation (*avatāra*):

Whenever there comes about a collapse of *dharma* and an uprising of *adharma*, then I emanate myself. For the protection of the good, and for the destruction of the evil-doers, for the purpose of re-establishing *dharma*, I become manifest in every age.

Though, he explains:

There is nothing in all the three worlds (*lokas*) that is duty for me, and nothing unobtained to be obtained.[2]

1. This book contains a wealth of information regarding *mantras* and kindred matters.
2. *Bhagavad Gītā*, iii, 20, 25; 22; iv, 7, 8. The idea of duty (*dharma*) is of vital import in the theory of right living propounded by Krishna in the *Gītā*. It is based on the theory of sacrifice, which states first that all beings are dependen t upon one another, and therefore one's duty is to use one's natural abilities (*sahaja karma*) and position in society (*jāti*) for the welfare of the world. When people in high places neglect their duty, the social situation becomes so bad that an Incarnation (*avatāra*) has to come. Each man does the best for himself when he uses his abilities for the welfare of the world. Further, he should use *his own* abilities and opportunities. 'Better is one's own duty, even if of poor quality, than the duty of another, even if well performed' (iii, 35; xviii, 45–7). As to the statement about desire or love (*kāma*): 'In all beings I am desire (*kāma*) which is not contrary to duty (*dharma*)' (vii, 11). In 'I am' the Divine is speaking, and the duty idea has to be linked up with the foregoing ideas about welfare of the world, and the principle of sacrifice. That is the way to perfection, and is proposed for those who want

Sir John Woodroffe's reference to the *mantra klīm* as *kāma bīja* is taken from the *Baradā Tantra*. I translate it as follows: 'K refers to the God of Love (*kāma*), otherwise Krishna, it is declared; l (indicates) Indra (the ruler of *swarga*, heaven); ī expresses satisfaction; and m is the giver of pleasure and pain.'

Sir John Woodroffe gives this explanation and also, from the same *Tantra*, the meanings of some other *mantras* of a similar kind, viz. *Hauṁ, Duṁ, Krīṁ, Hrīṁ, Shrīṁ, Aiṁ, Hūṁ, Gaṁ, Glauṁ, Kshrauṁ,* and *Strīṁ*.[1]

Similarly short and apparently meaningless *mantras* appear as the *bīja* (seed) *mantras* of the centres (*chakras*). It was necessary to list these when describing the centres or *chakras* in Chapter 8, but now they must be mentioned again with special reference to their effect as sounds. We may take them from below upwards, as the *hatha-yogi* or tantrist would do:

> The Basic Centre: *Laṁ*.
>
> The Pelvic Centre: *Vaṁ*.
>
> The Navel Centre: *Raṁ*.
>
> The Heart Centre: *Yaṁ*.
>
> The Throat Centre: *Haṁ*.
>
> The Brow Centre: *Oṁ*.

The first five of these *bījas*, as we have explained in our last chapter, are the *mantras* of the five 'elements' earth, water, fire, air, and ether respectively, with which the centres from the Basic Centre to the Throat Centre are respectively especially concerned. When meditating upon the deity and the power (*shakti*) in a *chakra*, the pronunciation, with meaning, of the seed-*mantra* will, it is considered, pro-

---

to and can rise to the standard proposed and thus become *buddhi-yogis* and *karma-yogis*. It is not for everybody, and there is no rebuke to those who do not at present want it (ii, 44). On the contrary, the wise man should not confuse the ignorant people who are attached to actions, but should encourage them to take pleasure in actions (iii, 26). This is in accordance with the general idea expounded at length in the later part of the *Gītā* that there are three grades of conduct or living, the sluggish, inert, gross (*tāmasa*), the active, restless, craving (*rājasa*), and the intelligent, orderly, sensible (*sāttwic*).

1. *The Garland of Letters*, pp. 245–9.

duce a good effect in the region governed by that *chakra*. But it must be 'with meaning', because the devotee's thought must be in tune with the character of the governing deity. The mere sound without the accompanying mental meaning will produce no effect.

The senses stimulated are, in order, counting upwards: smell, taste, sight, touch, and hearing – the sixth (the Brow Centre) having to do with the mental faculties. In our last chapter, the divinities in the *chakras* with their characteristics have been given. The devotee can meditate in any one of them for a particular purpose, but if aiming at the raising of Kundalinī would take all in turn, one after another, using the seed-*mantra* in each case. The terminal *ṁ* in each case is to be sounded exactly as in the case of *Oṁ*, which has been fully explained earlier in the present chapter.

Readers of Buddhist literature will no doubt be reminded, by these short words, of the well-known expression, '*Om mani padme hum*', *mani* being 'jewel', and *padme* 'in the lotus'. This is not a *mantra* but a statement and reminder. Although Gautama Buddha, the founder of Buddhism, spoke against the use of incantations and prayers and ceremonies his followers do often use fixed forms of words. These are generally regarded only as reminders, as in the case of the 'three refuges' (*tisarana*).

It is to be remembered, of course, that the word 'refuge' is not to be taken in the sense of dependence. Probably to call them 'resorts' would be better. I notice that Olcott's *Buddhist Catechism* speaks of them as the 'three guides'. Christmas Humphreys, President of the Buddhist Society, London, gives both the Pālī original and the translation as follows:

> Buddham saranam gacchami:
> (I go to the Buddha for Refuge).
>
> Dhammam saranam gacchami:
> (I go to the Doctrine for Refuge).
>
> Sangham saranam gacchami:
> (I go to the Order for Refuge).[1]

1. Humphreys, Christmas, *Buddhism* (Pelican Books), p. 242.

This is then repeated a second time and a third time by the devotees or aspirants for future enlightenment.

Another formula, having something of the character of a *mantra* as far as the mind is concerned, tells the simple religious aims of the southern Buddhists:

> Sabbapapassa akaranam,
> Kusalassa upasampada,
>
> Sa chitta pariyo dapanam—
> Etam Buddhanu sasanam.
>
> To cease from all sin,
> To get virtue,
> To cleanse one's own heart –
> This is the religion of the Buddhas.[1]

'This is quite a positive undertaking' is the reply to those who speak of Buddhism as passive. But Buddha definitely disapproved of any worship of deities or persons, including himself, and of ceremonies, advocating only what may be called the direct method for reaching 'the other shore'.

Buddha would not even permit anyone following his way to depend at all upon what is commonly called 'oneself', and for this also he provided the formula of the five *skandhas* or branches of our known being. These are given by Christmas Humphreys as follows:

The first is *Rupa*, form, shape, or body; in this sense the physical body, as including the organs of sense. The second is *Vedana*, which includes the feelings or sensations, whether pleasant, unpleasant, or neutral. The third is *Sanna*, comprising all perception or recognition, whether sensuous or mental. It is reaction to sense stimuli, described as 'awareness with recognition' or the idea which arises from such reaction. The fourth bundle, the *Sankharas*, includes all tendencies, mental and physical, the elements or factors in consciousness, all moral and immoral volitional activity, and the mental processes of discrimination and comparison between the ideas so brought into being. The fifth of the Skandhas, *Vinnana*, is as perishable and fleeting as the others. It is variously translated

1. Olcott, H. S., *A Buddhist Catechism*, p. 35.

as consciousness, mind, and mental powers, including the mental, moral, and physical predispositions.[1]

All these are compounded and impermanent. 'Impermanent are all component things.' 'Like the current of a river.' All of what man knows himself to be, taught Buddha, is impermanent or transitory. This bundle of five *skandhas* (branches) is like the old buggy in the story – one year its shafts were changed, another year its wheels, and so on – yet it continued to be called the same old buggy. The bundle goes on from life to life, but when *nirvāna* is achieved and accepted all five will be totally gone. Even the fifth *skandha* (or branch) is given the name *vinnana*, meaning consciousness or knowing, and that word comes from the Sanskrit *vi-jnā*, to perceive, observe, distinguish, know, and so refers to knowing something, and so indicates a subject-object relation, which is obviously of dependent origination and so is perishable.

Even when the Buddhists repeat the following formula they are not considered to be depending upon anything external, but only concentrating and adjusting their own minds to the Truth:

Gate,[2] *gate, paragate, parasangate, bodhi, swāhā.*

'Gone, gone, gone to the other shore, safely passed to that other shore, O Prajnā-pāramitā. So mote it be.'[3]

Still, the yogis maintained – except for the extreme right-wingers of *rāja-yoga* – that it is all right to use images and *mantras* as long as it is remembered that they are only temporary aids. And so the methods of Buddha, after a spectacular conquest of the country, gradually died away, because the aim of teachers like Sankarāchārya was just as 'beyond all this' as that of Buddha himself.

Therefore, among the Hindu yogis *mantra* is still very closely connected with devotion and worship (*bhakti-yoga*) because in *mantras* and their repetition (*japa*) only good

1. Humphreys, *op. cit.*, p. 94.
2. Pronounced as two syllables, ga-te, with 'e' as in 'grey'.
3. Translated freely from the *Mahā-prajnā-pāramitā-hridaya*, in Goddard, Dwight, *A Buddhist Bible*, New York (Dutton), p. 86.

things are to be embodied in the forms. The principle of *bhakti* is that the things we love and dwell upon we become. Hence the *mantras* of the gods and goddesses, who are powers and virtues, are effective, as they are names. That is why people sing hymns, and why in Indian villages there is constantly the singing of songs with the repetitions of names or praises (*bhajans*) which are set to pleasing music relating the sound to the thought and to that extent forming a mental home or habitat where the mind can rest in an upward-turned condition.

With respect to every *mantra* – as in the case of Western ceremonial – there must be *intent*, otherwise the words of a parrot or of a gramophone would carry the full power. When magical incantations are used, and there are blessings meant to help or curses meant to injure, we must consider them in two classes – those recited in the presence of the person to be affected, and those recited apart from him, and even secretly. In the former case there will be what may be called the musical effect, the tone and rhythm of the sound, in addition to the 'telepathic' effect. In this connexion it is well known that different kinds of music excite or depress different parts and functions of the body. Every word uttered in our hearing thus has some effect upon our minds and bodies. In the latter case the formula acts as a help to the sender of the blessing or curse, helping him to concentrate.

The subject of *mantras* could be carried further, into the domain of talismans and amulets. In this case certain objects have had blessings or curses pronounced over them, and even willed into them, as it were. To understand this feature of what to the layman appears to be a piece of magic, one must take into account that thoughts not only travel from one mind to another – like letters through the post – and impress the mind of the receiver according to his sensitiveness, but actually impress or cling to objects. Thus in some experiments which I conducted over fifty years ago, sets of blank cards were 'impressed', by concentrated thought, with pictures of various common objects. After the cards had been shuffled, and one had been put on a table near the sensitive subject or recipient (who was well blind-folded with a thick scarf) and out of sight of everybody present, the sensitive would describe the thought picture which had been impressed, and in this case was right every time. For this reason almost all people get some impressions of thought and feeling (emotion) from the objects they handle. Thus a book which has been well read will convey more than one new from the press.

In all these meditations only the good is desirable, and then only if loved. That is the universal solvent in all these meditations. If a little girl does not love her doll, she will not learn from it. All things that are loved awaken in us their own powers. If I love (or like) a chair I become a chair – a support and comfort – to others. If I love a wall, and observe that I do so because it is a protection against the weather, I become a wall – a protector of others. Straight things make me straight, and graceful things make me grace-ful, if I love them. The cat makes me a cat in such of its excellences as I admire and love; the dog, a dog; the saint, a saint; and so through all the variety and gamut of being. *Japa* and *mantra* are voluntary continuation of good com-panionship in the mind, and carry the benefits of remem-brance.

Closely related to the use of *mantras* is that of *yantras*. One is for hearing and the other for seeing. Just as the *mantra* is a sound-symbol of the deity concerned, so is the *yantra* a form-symbol. The *yantra* is the holder of the conceptual or formless deity as regards form. Thus we have three grades of repre-sentation, as it were – the divinity as expressed in abstract thought, then in sound, then in form. Then, just as a *mantra* expresses the deity in sound, so does the *yantra* in form. A devotee would go so far as to say that the divinity permeates the *mantra* and the *yantra*. All forms are thus permeated by their principles – what I have called their axes of creation. Our human form is clearly so, with its two sides, etc.

Yantric designs are often composed of various interlaced triangles and other figures having symbolic significance, innate or ultimate, as well as conventional. They offer great food for thoughtful meditation. Also they can be improved by being used or thought over, or by being blessed by a competent person – one who understands the *yantra*. Such *yantras* are sometimes called *mandalas* when they are included in a frame, usually circular. They are much used in tantric circles and in Tibet. Common objects are full of broken bits of *yantras*, so to speak, but if an entire form were perfectly coordinate and integrated it would be a *yantra*.

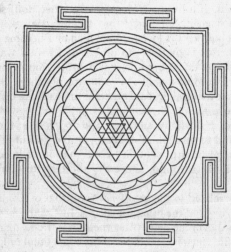

So the *yantra* is something that can hold the mind to a form with some basic guidance, and the mind contemplating that form and including all the designs it contains may easily pass along to the integral concept. Therefore the example that is depicted in our illustration, though not an exact representation of any particular one in use, can give an idea of the use as well as the general appearance of a typical *yantra*.[1] It can be gazed at with a varying combinative look-

1. The forms of the *yantra* of Kundalinī are depicted on the covers of Arthur Avalon's books, and the *Saundarya-Laharī* translated by the

ing which could ultimately include all the possible groupings and formations – much as in a less organized way one can see pictures (one's own creations, but even intuitive creations if the mind is intent and quiet enough) in the glowing embers of a fire or in a cloud.

The more perfectly designed a *yantra* is for a particular divinity, the more fully will its axes of creation disclose the varieties of involvement permeated by the abstract idea of that divinity. Each involved part is a halting-place in manifestation for the temporary dwelling of the contemplating mind.

Specimens of different kinds of *mantras* have been given in this chapter. One more has to be mentioned – what is called the *Ajapā Gāyatrī*. It is *ajapā* (not repeated) because it is not voluntarily recited, but takes place day and night, with only occasionally a little notice by ourselves. It is our ordinary breathing. It is a *mantra* because it comes in with sound of *sa* and goes out with the sound of *ha*, little as we may notice it. It cannot be regarded as a *mantra* in the strict sense of the word, because a *mantra* must have a meaning or conscious intention, whereas this goes on normally 21,600 times in the day and night, say all the books, without intent. The two sounds put together, however, do present a meaning.

After the disciple has been taught by his *guru* in the *Chhāndogya Upanishad* that 'Thou art That' (*Tat twam asi*) he can, if he has realized that he himself is of the nature of That, not This, spontaneously say *So'ham*.[1] The exact meaning of these words is first *Sah*, which means He or That, and then *aham*, I am. In accordance with the requirements of euphony of the Sanskrit language the *ah* of *sah* becomes *o* and then the vowel *a* of *aham* is dropped. For the full yogi, every breath, every heartbeat also, expresses and declares the Unity.

Pandit R. Anantakrishna Shāstri and Shri Karrā Rāmamūrthy, Madras (Ganesh & Co.). The latter contains illustrations of *yantras* and their parts with explanations, including many of the *yantras* of the mantric syllables, *klīm*, etc.

1. Strangely coming near to our phrase 'So I am!'

This could be equally stated with the words reversed, and then we would have *hansa*, which means a swan. The swan is a religious symbol – the bird of time. It is on the wing and indicates the manifesting Brahman (*Shabdabrahman*). Breathing is a time process and, in fact, both in the mind and in the body, we live 'on the wing', and it is almost the first lesson in practical philosophy to recognize and accept this fact. Some of the yogis who are somewhat advanced are in fact entitled *hansas* (swans) and *paramahansas* (superior swans). There is another legend about this bird. It is able to take the milk and leave the water in a mixture of the two, and in a similar way the yogi in this degree knows how to extract the soul's benefit from the mixture of experience which constitutes our lives.

Somewhat akin to the same idea is the meaning embodied in the first four stages of the upward way. The candidate really sets his foot on this path when he learns not to seek any settled condition in material things. In this sense he gives up regarding himself as resting on anything, or wishing to have anything forever. He then is called a *Parivrājaka*, a wanderer. In this condition he may feel a little lost until he discovers an equilibrium in himself, whereupon he reaches the second stage and is called *Kutīchaka*, the builder of a hut. In the third stage he becomes the *Hansa*, the swan already mentioned, in which he does not concern himself with an inner resting-place or basis, but is busy getting the good out of everything (the milk out of the water), until he finds, as Emerson put it:

> Every day brings a ship,
> Every ship brings a word;
> Well for those who have no fear,
> Looking seaward, well assured
> That the word the vessel brings
> Is the word they wish to hear.

Now he is beyond liking and disliking, for he gets the good out of everything. There is no longer any antagonism. He is at peace with the world, even when the world is not at peace with him. Now, again, as Emerson saw: 'To the poet, to the philosopher, to the saint, all things are friendly and sacred, all events profitable, all days holy, all men divine; for the eye is fastened on the life, and slights the circumstance.' After that there is only the fourth stage, which we may leave to be sought rather than described. He has nothing more to learn – from the world.

CHAPTER 12

THE YOGA OF THE *BHAGAVAD GĪTĀ*

THE *Bhagavad Gītā* is regarded in India as the greatest compendium of religious inspiration – devotional, philosophical, ethical, and moral. It is well known in the Western world also, through perhaps a hundred translations into English and various European languages. It is not so well known that every chapter in it is entitled a form of yoga, such as 'The Yoga of Action', 'The Yoga of Knowledge', 'The Yoga of Devotion', 'The Yoga of the Royal Science and the Royal Mystery'. Therefore an extract of its yoga methods must find place here.

First of all, it offers many brief definitions and descriptions of yoga, for example:

Yoga is equilibrium in success and failure (ii, 48).
Yoga is skilful living among activities (ii, 50).
Yoga is an ancient science, revived by Shrī Krishna (iv, 3).
Yoga is the supreme secret of life (iv, 3).
Yoga is a producer of the greatest felicity (v, 2).
Yoga is serenity (vi, 3).
Yoga is non-attachment (vi, 4).
Yoga is the destroyer of pain (vi, 17).
Yoga is separation from pain (vi, 23).
Yoga is effected by self-control (vi, 36).
Yoga uses concentration (viii, 12).
Yoga is attained by contemplation (ii, 53).
Yoga practice is for self-purification (vi, 12).

Again, different kinds or methods of yoga are mentioned, e.g.:

Sānkhya-yoga – yoga by science.
Buddhi-yoga – yoga by wisdom.
Ātma-yoga – yoga of the Self.
Karma-yoga – yoga by action.
Sannyāsa-yoga – yoga by renunciation.

Various terms associated with yoga practices found in the *Gītā* are used with the same meaning as the same terms in the *Yoga Sūtras* of Patanjali. Such are *dhāranā*, meaning concentration, *dhyāna*, meaning meditation, and *samādhi*, meaning profound contemplation, all found in the *Gītā*.

In view of the fact that the *Bhagavad Gītā* is a scripture of yoga, and calls itself such, we will now give a brief survey of the teaching in each of the chapters, omitting only the first chapter, which merely describes the circumstances in which Shrī Krishna gave the teaching, and how the mental depression of his disciple Arjuna in those circumstances called it forth.

Chapter 2. The teacher tells the disciple that he should not be grieved by death. He teaches that the owner of the body (*dehī*) will exist after death and existed before birth and, in fact, never did not exist or will not exist. This spirit is the real man, and takes body after body. The body is temporary and is as it were a garment. Pleasures and pains are temporary and should be taken as they come.

All this Krishna describes as scientifically known (*sānkhya*), because in his day these matters were taken to be matters well established by what would today be called the psychical observations and researches of many yogis.

This is not left as a mere negative or consoling doctrine. The Teacher says that scientific knowledge is not enough. In modern terms, knowledge of facts does not tell us what to do. There must be the application of it to the benefit of the continuing life. There is such a thing as wisdom (*buddhi*), which is knowing the life and its needs, and so giving proper value to the things and using them for that purpose. He goes so far as to call the endeavour to make this wisdom constant and never to lose sight of it in any circumstances *buddhi-yoga*.

This is not different from Patanjali's yoga, for he also puts in the forefront what we may call his ten commandments,[1] without which all attempts to realize the real man will be ineffective. People who have not these virtues are engulfed

1. See Chapter 3.

in desires for bodily pleasures and self-satisfaction, which constitutes a bondage to laziness (*tamas*), or excitement (*rajas*), or orderliness (*sattwa*), which are qualities of the environment, and of the body, not of the real man. Such people want a pleasant heaven after death, but the *buddhi-yogi* takes his circumstances as they come, good or bad, pleasant or unpleasant, and does what he can for the benefit of all concerned. His buddhic wisdom gives a new motive for action, and this makes him a practical man, a *karma-yogi*.

This is not inconsistent with having times dedicated to meditation, but the ideal condition will be reached when in the midst of all circumstances he is able to have the wisdom and insight reached at the times of deepest meditation. Then he will perform actions in union with the divine, and not disturbed by success or failure, fully attentive to the work of the moment and not worrying about whether he will succeed or fail. He is not working for results, but to do his best. And his wisdom will not be confused if he practises *samādhi*, that is, meditation and deep contemplation.

In practice, this means that he will be free from anxiety, fear, anger, pride, and attachment to things, and will quite naturally acquire a great deal of control of his body and his mind.

Chapter 3. Shrī Krishna states that from ancient times he taught two paths – yoga by knowledge (*jnāna-yoga*) and yoga by action (*karma-yoga*). The former, he says, is the method of the followers of the *sānkhya*; the latter that of the yogis. Whenever he says yogis he means *buddhi-yogis*, unless otherwise stated. We may say with respect to the former, which gives a study and classification of all things, that its two greatest classes are (1) the real man (*purusha*) and (2) everything else, all included in the material (*prakriti*) in the widest sense of the term, including even the human mind. One may say, in this regard, that if one saw with absolute clearness the distinction between *purusha* and *prakriti* one would know the *purusha* properly, which is the goal of yoga.

The Teacher now expounds right action. Actions done

with desire for bodily pleasure or self-satisfaction bind a man to circumstances, but actions done as sacrifice (*yajna*) do not attach one to things and thus make one dependent upon them. Sacrifice, he says, means nourishing one another. All things are related in a great system of mutual support, so one should recognize this principle and always act accordingly. But suppose a man has a perception of the real Self (*purusha* or *ātmā*) and that is his real interest, he can withdraw from action. He has finished, and has no desire for reincarnation or for heaven. As he is still alive, he has what is called actionless action (*naishkarmya karma*). His actions are now pure duty, and are done with body and mind, while he is conscious of being the real man. He performs actions purely for the welfare of the world, knowing how people follow examples, and knowing that people in general are acting with desire. In this he is only in line with the example of the Incarnate Lord, without which, coming into the world from time to time, people would not have a leading in the path of duty. This is where religious devotion comes in.

The yogi at this stage realizes that in the world each thing acts – action, not only substance, is part of its being. Each acts according to its own nature, and some of them are mainly *tāmasic* (inert), some are mainly *rājasic* (energetic and even restless), and some are (*sāttwic*) orderly and methodical. They are all just the forces of Nature, but the Self or real man has no bodily action and no mental action – nothing in fact to which we could apply any conception of action, without bringing in a presumption (*adhyāsa*) which would block our further vision or realization. One may say that these three qualities of Nature's appear to agree with the constituents of Nature with which the modern scientist is always concerned, namely, matter, energy, and law.

In doing action, or one's duty, the Teacher says there are to be no external standards. It is doing one's own duty, however unexciting, that is most beneficial. Imitation is dangerous. Desire and anger are to be discouraged. The great thing to admire and serve is the supreme Self. It is greater than *buddhi*. *Buddhi* is greater than mere mentality, and that is greater than the senses, which, however, are never-theless great, but That which is mentionable only as That is above all. This chapter is called the yoga of action, and teaches both understanding and doing.

It seems necessary to bring out a little more decisively the meaning of *karma-yoga* – a path followed by so many ad-herents to the *Gītā* teaching. When the actions of daily life are permeated by the buddhic devotion to life, those actions become yoga, *karma-yoga*. Every action can thus be yoga. Washing dishes with love is yoga. The actions going on in a dish-washing machine are not. If a doctor performs a sur-gical operation merely thinking of the money he will get, it is not yoga. To do it from a sense of duty would not be yoga. But if it is done for the welfare of the patient it is yoga. Many people's karma is thus black; the true yogi's karma is white; most people's actions are shall we say grey.

Joy goes with the whiteness of the *karma-yoga*, because there is more life in it. Incidentally, much of the modern bringing-up of children is very stultifying and boring to them in this respect. Modern schooling which takes the children away from home duties is sometimes almost tragic. If the children are all the time recipients, and are deprived of the experience of the enjoyment of mutual help, there is bound to be boredom which no amount of rich toys or cul-tivation of self-esteem can compensate.

Such is the *karma-yoga* of the *Gītā*. It does not put 'good deeds' and 'bad deeds' in the limelight, but the wisdom that is love permeated by understanding. This is also not 'unin-telligent love'. This theme, so emphasized in Chapters 2 and 3 of the *Gītā*, is continued in Chapter 4.

Chapter 4. It is real knowledge, Shrī Krishna now says, to observe and realize the part played in Nature and life by action. Doing so you will come to 'my' state – doing the actionless action while living in the world. In this one does not desire results. One may, perhaps, make a comparison. Someone asks: 'If one gives up desires for bodily pleasure and self-satisfaction, will there not be a slackening of efforts?' The answer is, 'Not if *buddhi* is awake. It provides the new motive.' Then comes the question: 'Suppose that *buddhi* is also given up. Will there not then be no motive?' The answer is, 'Not if there is the divine motive, as exemplified by the divine Incarnation (*avatāra*) who acts without anything to gain. It is pure love that is exemplified. One can see the idea in the life of Jesus, who, when asked what he wanted his questioners to do, answered, 'I want you to love one another *as* I have loved you'. This is not action. It does not change. Body and mind do the actions under this rule or law. Just so, Jesus did not impose rules, but gave people something to do, viz. love.

The man is then described as pleased with whatever comes. This equanimity (*samatwa*) is of the mind. It is really the philosophical attitude which should be the outcome of the *sānkhya* (scientific) knowledge or belief. It may seem that bodily pains are lessened by it, but that is somewhat illusory. The fact is that usually our bodily pains are felt more acutely because we add an intense concentration of mind upon them, and also add an emotional pain. The trouble may be real, but thus men make another trouble, and so there is double trouble and quite often the second trouble is worse than the first. The emotional equanimity arising from philosophical understanding is what is aimed at. It is not intended that there should be passive endurance or resignation. When there is equanimity one can tackle the real problem with all one's faculties. First of all, then, the searchlight of self-pity, disappointment, and even perhaps anger and hate is turned out, and secondly the man is at his best to deal with the real pain or trouble. Equanimity becomes non-antagonism to any situation that arises, and that is practical realism.

This is probably the best place to consider the three chief verbs in our life – to be, to do, and to have. The aspirant who watches himself will find that he is only interested in being. Is it that he wants a nice house? Really he wants to *be* comfortable, and if it is a matter of keeping up with the Joneses, or even of surpassing them, he wants self-satisfaction, and if he too is thwarted he may go to a psychologist who tries to help him to find a suitable or attainable niche and be satisfied, whereas if he had gone to a yogi he would have given him equanimity and set him free from niches.

The idea of this central philosophy of the *Gītā* was somewhat understood by the Stoics, as Epictetus showed when he said, 'There is only one thing for which God has sent me into the world and that is to perfect my own nature in every sort of strength, and there is nothing in all the world which I cannot use for that purpose.' Inwardly, then, the role is equanimity, and outwardly usefulness. If there are exercises, it is to establish and maintain these in both body and mind.

When at or near this stage, Krishna says that men perform many different actions of sacrifice – following in their own way the aims of perfection or perfect action, partly as duty, and partly as devotion to the Incarnation or perhaps rather to what it exemplifies. Krishna enumerates some of these, and then comes the statement in one of his key verses that the offering of knowledge is greater than any material offering, because all acts have their fulfilment in knowledge – clearly meaning philosophical and religious knowledge, for he further states that this can be learned by devotion, inquiry, and service, and from those who already know it.

Then, says Krishna, you will see that everything is divine, and knowledge will remove all faults and clear away the dependence upon particular outside things.

Chapter 5. This chapter is called the 'Yoga of Renunciation'. This is the renunciation of action in the sense that the yogi realizes that the actions are done by the mind and the body and the many energies of the outside world. Riding in a motor-car, one may see clearly that it is the car that is running along the road, not oneself. Even moving the controls, it is thought that guides the hand or foot. One is not doing it. What it is that has caused this relation between thought and hand is unknown. Carry the argument a step further – one can say that even the thought is an inner machine, and there is oneself behind that, and then care must be taken not to attribute to the oneself action such as that of the body or of the mind. That owner of the body or as some put it dweller in the body must not be confused with the mind.

As we have seen, we have to go beyond that, the whole mind being only the inner instrument (*antahkarana*). Then, as the *Gītā* puts it, the yogi thinks, 'I do not do anything', even while seeing, hearing, touching, smelling, tasting, walking, sleeping, breathing, evacuating, holding. Krishna maintains 'The organs move among the objects of sense'. Yet the business is done by that Ātmā who is with the Brahman (God), though without action. All the objects of the world are 'fruit of action' (*karma-phala*). It is all the actionless action of the Brahman. That is the unit necessary to both variety and harmony.

So the yogi acts only for 'self-purification', not for getting something. He renounces that, and strives to put all his action in the Divine, making it the actionless action which has its own illumination, beyond desire for things or for knowledge. *That* (not this) is what he values; it is his very Self. 'He is the happy man; he rejoices within; he is illuminated within.' 'He goes to the nirvana of Brahman.'

At the end of this chapter some practical hints for meditation are given:

Having put the external contacts outside and (having made) the gaze even between the eyebrows, (and) having made equal the in and out breaths travelling within the nose, (and) with senses, *manas* and *buddhi* controlled, the aspirant, with liberation as his chief aim, his desire, fear, and anger being gone – it is even he who is always free.

Having known me, the enjoyer of *yajna* and *tapas*, the great lord (*īshwara*) of all worlds, the friend of all beings – he goes to peace (*shānti*).[1]

Chapter 6. When the man is seeking yoga, we are now told, he will of course undertake various actions and be involved in them, but when he is really 'mounted on yoga' he will have no attachment to either objects or actions. He stands above illusion. To him all things have the same value – earth, a stone, gold. He has the same buddhic outlook to-

1. *Bhagavad Gītā*, v, 27–9.

wards friends, enemies, strangers, neutrals, haters, saints, sinners. He is poised in cold and heat, pleasure and pain, respect and contumely.

Some more practical hints are now given:

The yogi should practise meditation always on the Self, sitting in private, alone, having himself and his thoughts controlled – without expectation, without grasping.

Having settled in a clean place on a firm seat of his own, not too high and not too low, which has some kusha grass, a furry skin, and a cloth upon it – there, having made the mind one-pointed, with the senses and thoughts and actions controlled, having sat on the seat, he should practise yoga (meditation) for the purification of himself.

Holding body, head, and the back of the neck properly (*samam*), unmoving and steady, and having (next) looked in front of his nose[1] without seeing in any direction, being himself quieted, with fears all gone, steady in observance of Brahma-conduct, having poised the mind with me as (its) thought, let him sit, united, with me as his Beyond (*para*).

The yogi, with mind controlled, always meditating thus on the Self, arrives at my state, the nirvanic ultimate, which is peace.

But yoga is not for the excessive eater, and not for one who avoids food too intently, and not for one addicted to excessive sleep, also not to wakefulness.

Yoga becomes the destroyer of pain for one whose food and recreations are appropriate, whose efforts in actions are appropriate, whose sleeping and waking are appropriate.

When the controlled mind stays only on the Self, without longing for all objects of desire – then one is called united (*yukta*).[2]

Thus, Krishna continues, the yogi becomes like a lamp standing where there is no wind. Controlled by the practice of yoga, the lower mind becomes quiet. Seeing the self in the Self – the consciousness is directly conscious of itself – the yogi rejoices. He does not waver from the truth, and now he is not moved even by heavy pain. He sees the Self, and in his meditation he thinks of nothing else. Having found it, being established in the unity, he sees the same Self everywhere and lives in the Divine, whatever he is doing.

1. The front of the nose is held by some to mean with eyes unfocused, by others between the eyebrows, and with some at the tip of the nose.
2. *Bhagavad Gītā*, vi, 10–18.

Arjuna, the disciple, now sees before him what appears to be a difficult task. He points out the difficulty of controlling the mind and also wonders what happens if the aspirant fails to achieve the desired state or even falls by the wayside. Krishna has already said that from whatever cause the unsteady mind wanders off, the disciple should hold it back and lead it into the power of the *ātmā*. And the power of *ātmā* is the influence of the Self. When the Self is seen even a little, its appeal or pull is tremendous. That is what makes the philosophical or metaphysical vision or insight, to which the disciple should resort again and again. However, Shrī Krishna is endlessly patient. He says:

Certainly the restless mind (*manas*) is difficult to control, but by practice (*abhyāsa*) and uncolouredness (*vairāgya*) it is controlled.[1]

Practice (*abhyāsa*) and uncolouredness (*vairāgya*) are the same two words given by Patanjali in the *Yoga Sūtras* as the basis of the practice he lays down.[2]

In reference to Arjuna's second question, about failure, Shrī Krishna replies in detail:

Having reached the worlds of those who have done good, and having dwelt (there) very many years, he who fell from yoga is born in a pure and fortunate house. Or he even comes into a family of wise yogis, though a birth such as this is very hard to obtain in this world. There he obtains the buddhic attainments of his previous incarnation and thence again strives for full accomplishment.[3]

It is generally considered among Hindu scholars that the first six chapters contain the philosophical teachings of the *Gītā*, while the next six contain the devotional, and the last six contain information of a more detailed or practical kind. This sixth chapter was called the *Dhyāna yoga* by the famed commentator Shankarāchárya. The reader will have noticed how it aims at the deepest philosophical insight.

Chapter 7. In this seventh chapter, Krishna begins by

1. *Bhagavad Gītā*, vi, 35.   2. See Chapter 4.   3. *Bhagavad Gītā*, vi, 40–3.

naming the constituents of the external world – five material and three of the mind – but only in order to instruct the disciple as to what to discard or eliminate in seeking to know the divine Being and the divine Self. Eight constituents of the lower nature (*prakriti*) are listed, viz. earth, water, fire, air, ether, mind (*manas*), wisdom or valuation (*buddhi*), and the individuality (*ahankāra*). Beyond these, says Krishna, speaking as Incarnation, there is another nature, my life-element, by which all this world is maintained.

He then refers to himself as the source of the distinguishing perfection of every excellent thing – the light of the sun and moon, the sacred syllable (*Om*) among words, the good odour in the earth, the brightness of fire, the vitality in all beings, the strength of the strong, etc. 'I am not in them, but they are in me.' This indicates that all perfections represent axes of growth which have their origin beyond mind and body. This knowledge is a stimulus to devotion to That.

As to the devotees, there are four kinds, who are all good people – he who is distressed; he who desires knowledge; he who seeks wealth; and he who has knowledge. The last is best. He is the *Mahātmā* (great soul or self), who declares, from knowledge, that Brahman is all. He understands the unborn and unchanging, the Beyond.

The good, their sins ended, their minds free from confusion, their resolves firm, 'are devoted to me'. These, striving for liberation from the worlds of decay and death, devoted 'to me', know Brahman, the oversoul (*adhyātmā*), and entire action, along with the material things (*adhibhūta*), the life side (*adhidaiva*), and the principle of sacrifice (*adhiyajna*). 'And they know me at the time of death.'

This thinking of Brahman at the time of death is regarded as a very important matter, and the listing of six items just mentioned, to be distinguished from one another, and to be seen at work in our lives is the best means to realize the glorious presence. When that glorious presence is found, its raying is seen to be the basis of all glories (*vibhūtis*), and therefore it is stated that all beings are *from* That, and they are also *in* That, inasmuch as they could not exist without that presence. A crude illustration of this is a pot, and the clay it is made from. And if it is said that we find that forms made by mind (all the tools, inventions, machines, clothing, houses, etc., and even, though less directly, the limbs and organs of living bodies) are independent when once they are made, still it must be added that that ability to retain themselves is also something derived from the supreme presence.

Chapter 8 begins with a brief description of the six things listed at the end of Chapter 7, and just as one must be able to distinguish the five kinds of ideas – according to Patanjali's yoga[1] – in order to be mentally sane, so one must be able to distinguish these six things in order to be philosophically aware of the glorious presence. Krishna now defines them:

(*a*) Brahman is the indestructible, the supreme.

(*b*) The self-existent is the oversoul (*adhyātmā*).

(*c*) The emanation or ray which causes the rise of existing forms is action (*karma*).

It may here be explained that 'entire action' means the whole course of cause and effect, every effect becoming a cause in its turn. Its meaning also includes the three kinds of action – that of the body, that of the mind, and that beyond – the actionless action already studied. Here perhaps it may also be explained that when a person receives the result of his own action, he will give a response and it is desirable that it should be from all three levels. Inasmuch as there is some actionless action there is an *influence* of the *ātmā*, affecting the mind from within or from above as an intuition or illumination. Actions emanating from that state do not produce an effect upon the doer, because this doer is an actionless doer, beyond the sequence, and free – in a word, divine, self-existent, uninfluenced.

(*d*) The material side of things (*adhibhūta*) is the perishable or objective nature, what is acted upon.

(*e*) The subjective nature is the life-side (*adhidaiva*), the whole mind, with its will, feeling, and thought, corresponding to *ahankāra*, *buddhi*, and *manas*.

1. *Yoga Sūtras*, i, 5–11.

(*f*) As to the principle of sacrifice (*adhiyajna*), Shrī Krishna calls it 'me here in the body'.

All acts of sacrifice, it will be remembered, are acts for mutual benefit, not for personal desire. Mutual benefit is the rule of Nature, and those who have not yet come to the point where they respond to this principle (on account of the awakening of *buddhi*) are compelled to submit to it by outside pressure (by the law of karma). But a person such as Krishna or – to turn to the great Western example – such as Jesus, who, because of love (which is inherent as the active side of *buddhi*), gives his time, knowledge, and energy entirely to the welfare of others, instead of to personal pleasures, is a living sacrifice. Jesus said, 'Whosoever would be my disciple must take up his cross daily and follow me', no doubt meaning follow his way of life. Thus he gives up his personal selfish life and discovers 'the life everlasting'. And surely the word cross, being referred to as taken up daily, must mean the business and efforts of daily life, which are to be carried on in the right spirit. And that right spirit is no less than God here in the flesh.

At this point Shrī Krishna reverts again to the idea of remembering the divine at the time of death. This must surely refer to the state of mind at the time of death. Has a person or has he not a realization of the 'actionless' before and at that time? It cannot be mere words that are indicated by 'remembering me'. If he has, then comes the statement that when he 'leaves the body, and goes forth remembering definitely me (*mām eva*), without doubt he goes to my (state of) being'.[1] If not, then he goes to that which he thinks about.[2]

We come now to some more practical statements, having reference to this 'time of forthgoing'. First let us notice the statements that he leaves the body and goes forth:

Having his mind unwandering at the time of death, united by devotion and by the strength of yoga, having well placed (his) life-breath (*prāna*) in the middle of the eyebrows, he goes to that divine real man (*purusha*) beyond.[3]

1. *Bhagavad Gītā*, viii, 5–8. 2. *ibid.*, vii, 23. 3. *ibid.*, viii, 10.

And:

Having controlled all the doors, and having kept the mind in the heart, (and being) established in yogic concentration, pronouncing '*Om*', the One-syllabled Brahman, keeping on remembering me, he who (thus) dies, giving up the body, goes to the supreme goal.[1]

'Between the two eyebrows' indicates the Brow Centre (*ājnā chakra*) which has been studied in our Chapter 9.

Then the Teacher says:

Who remembers me constantly, always having his conscious attention (*chetas*) upon no other – for that constantly united yogi I am easy to reach.

Having come to me, the Mahatmas do not again obtain birth, which is the non-eternal place of pain, having gone to the supreme attainment. (All) worlds, (even) up to the abode of Brahmā, are (worlds of) returning (to birth), but (for one) having come to me there is no birth again.[2]

Chapters 9, 10, 11, and 12 are pre-eminently devotional discourses. They do not lack philosophic background, which is entirely of the kind so far described. Therefore the devotion is not emotional, but is the result of deep philosophical insight.

Perhaps we may again refer to the predominantly Western religion and remind the reader that Jesus gave two commandments: (1) To love God and (2) to love one's neighbour. When men love their neighbours it is clear that they are thinking of the neighbour's benefit, not their own. This is the nature of love. When men love God, must there not be the same kind of devotion? This devotion must be an intense gratitude, and that in its turn must depend upon a clear experience. How shall a man love something that he does not know? Hence the devotion spoken of must imply knowledge.

The entire contents of the chapters of the *Gītā* now under review are bent to the task of helping the disciple to get a more complete and accurate idea of the deity. They thus form a sort of prolonged meditation and constitute material

1. *ibid.*, viii, 12, 13.   2. *ibid.*, viii, 15, 16.

for meditation – many meditations upon the qualities and greatness of various classes of things and beings of archetypal value are indicated, and the series ends up with Arjuna's vision of the universal form.

The Divine does not ask for rich and expensive ceremonies and gifts:

He who offers to me with devotion a leaf, a flower, a fruit (or) water – that, offered with devotion by the striving self, I absorb. Whatever you eat, whatever you offer, whatever you give, whatever austerity (*tapas*) you do, do that as offering to me.[1]

Also he does not aim at attracting the great:

I am the same towards all beings. There is none repugnant to me, nor favourite, but those who serve me with devotion – they are in me, and in them also I am. Even if one of very bad conduct serves me, not serving another, he should be considered good, since he is well-determined. Quickly he becomes a *dharmic* self (and) goes to the eternal peace.[2]

At the end of Chapter 10, after enumerating many glories he explains:

Whatever is the seed in all beings, that I am, and there is not anything that can be without me, either moving or unmoving.

There is no end to my divine glories. What I have declared is only illustrative of the extent of my glories.

Whatever is glorious, orderly, illustrious, or great – understand that it has origin in a share of my splendour.

But what is the use of more of this knowledge to you? Having established this entire universe with one share, I stand.[3]

The term share may be explained a little. It implies no separation of a created object from its creator and no difference of nature. As Emerson said: 'There is no bar or wall in the human soul where man the effect leaves off and God the cause begins.' The Sanskrit word for share used in this verse, and in verse xv, 7, is *ansha*. This definitely means a share. If something is shared out (as e.g. a piece of cake) every portion has the same nature. Such is the creation of man by God, according to the *Gītā*.

1. *ibid.*, ix, 26.   2. *ibid.*, ix, 29, 30.   3. *ibid.*, x, 39–42.

The last of this group of chapters describes the devotee. The following descriptive verses are especial favourites with thousands upon thousands of devotional people who follow what is called the *bhakti-yoga*.

Without hatred for any being, friendly, compassionate, without possessiveness, without egotism, equal in pain and pleasure, forgiving, contented, always having yoga, self-controlled, firmly purposeful and with *manas* and *buddhi* intent upon me – he, who is my devotee, is to me beloved.

He from whom the world does not shudder away, and who does not shudder away from the world, and who is free from the up-rushing of sensuous enthusiasms, anger, and fear – he is to me beloved.

He who is not looking for something (for his pleasure or happiness) is pure, industrious, impartial, untroubled (by what happens), and who has given up all undertakings – he, who is my devotee, is to me beloved.

He who does not exult, is not hostile, does not grieve, does not long (for anything), (and) has given up attachment to the lovely and the unlovely – he, having *bhakti*, is to me beloved.

The same to foe and friend, and likewise when respected and disrespected, and the same in cold and heat and pleasure and pain, (and) free from attachments, equal when reproached or praised, silent, contented with whatever is, without a home, with steady purpose – (that) man, having *bhakti*, is to me beloved.

But those who devote themselves to this deathless way of life, as (now) declared, having wealth of faith, with me as supreme – those devotees are to me exceedingly beloved.[1]

Chapters 13 to 18 of the *Gītā* give some details concerning the philosophical doctrines already expounded. Chapter 13 deals with the 'Yoga of the Distinction between the Field and the knower of the Field', or Matter and Spirit. It describes the Knower as the Supreme Brahman (*parabrahman*), as standing in the world, pervading everything, having all the functions of the senses without any organs, being outside and inside all beings, not divided among beings but standing as though divided, maintaining all beings, and absorbing and producing them. It is called the light of all lights

1. *ibid.*, xii, 13–20.

beyond the darkness. Whatever being is born, it is explained, is due to the junction of the knower of the field with the field.

There is in each being that ruler (*ishwara*) – the same inner ruler in every case, actionless while the material (field) does all the actions. The combinations of the three qualities of Nature (*tamas, rajas,* and *sattwa*) are the material basis of all things. The distribution and predominances of these three – inertia, mobility or restlessness, and harmony or orderliness – is detailed in Chapter 14. The *sattwic* condition of the body and mind is the only one of the three which can permit of liberation, for the other two are concerned with worldly attachments of enjoyment (*bhoga*) or self-satisfaction (*aishwarya*) or with possessiveness, desire, and aversion, or egotism.

Chapter 15 takes up the simile of a tree, with, however, its roots above and its branches below. The disciple will cut this tree down with the axe of non-attachment, saying: 'I go even to that original spirit from whom the ancient manifestation was extended.'[1]

The teacher now tells how the situation for each one of us has come about:

A share of myself, having become an eternal living being in the world of living beings, attracts the sense-organs, of which *manas* is the sixth, which are situated in Nature.

(This) master (*ishwara*), who (thus) obtains a body and who also goes beyond it (at death), having grasped these (senses) goes his way, just as the wind (takes) scents from their resting-places.

Having governed the ear, the eye, the organs of touch and taste and smell, and the *manas,* he makes use of the objects of sense.

The deluded do not perceive him (thus) joined with the qualities (*gunas*), whether he is departing or staying still, or enjoying (the senses). They see, whose eye is knowledge.

Yogis, striving, also see him, instated in themselves. The inattentive, who have not disciplined themselves even though striving, do not see him.[2]

Chapter 16 lists the good qualities of human character,

1. *ibid.,* xv, 4.   2. *ibid.,* xv, 7–11.

and then the bad qualities of those who yield themselves to desire and pride. In Chapter 17 the subject of the three qualities of Nature (*gunas*) is taken up again, and there is a list of them showing themselves in three kinds of faith and worship, three kinds of food, three kinds of sacrifice, austerity, etc. Pure (*sattwic*) foods are listed as those which increase vitality, bodily harmoniousness, strength, health, pleasure, and bodily gratification – juicy, oily, firm, and heartening. People who inflict upon themselves fierce austerities are severely condemned. The chapter concludes with the *mantra* '*Om Tat Sat*', described in Chapter 11.

Finally, Chapter 18, called the 'Yoga of Renunciation' (*sannyāsa*), says the renunciation means not renunciation of actions, but renunciation of desire for the fruit of actions, and this means that there will still be three kinds of actions in the life of the renouncer (*sannyāsī*), namely gift (*dāna*), voluntary sacrifice (*yajna*), and strictness of life (*tapas*).

The question of causation in actions is then taken up, and it is stated that five things contribute to the result in every case, viz. the man himself, his body, the tools and limbs he uses, the functions employed, and lastly fate or the unseen. The last is always expected to play a part, so that, as Burns said, 'The best laid schemes of mice and men aft gang agley', and on the other hand the bungler may have 'luck'. The effect of the last of these ingredients has long been woven into the Hindu character, so that people are not so surprised or disappointed or distressed as the Westerner when things go wrong, or unduly elated when they go right. There is also no resentment about it, for the unexpected and uncalculated is credited to the effects of past actions (the law of karma), whether good or bad.

People are classified according to character and occupation (caste), and an oft-repeated formula is adducted:

Better is one's own *dharma*, (though) imperfect, than the *dharma* of another, well performed. In doing the activity marked out by one's own form of existence one acquires no fault.[1]

1. *ibid.*, xviii, 47.

Then comes the climax, the statement that he whose *buddhi* is unattached to anything, who is self-governed and has given up longing, attains by *sannyāsa* to the supreme perfection beyond all activity. 'Always doing actions, and resorting to me, by my grace he obtains the eternal unchanging goal.'[1]

The Teacher concludes, leaving his pupil perfectly free, saying that the deepest knowledge has now been communicated, and ending: 'Having reflected upon it completely, then act as you will. Can it be that this has been heard by you, O Arjuna, with one-pointed attention? Can it be that your confusion, caused by ignorance, has been dispelled?'[2]

1. *ibid.*, xviii, 56.   2. *ibid.*, xviii, 63, 72.

CHAPTER 13

THE BASIC PHILOSOPHY OF YOGA[1]

Now we will have a course of instruction in yoga, which is the control of ideas in the mind. When this is done the conscious being is in his own proper state; otherwise he is conditioned by the ideas. There is always a judging of ideas as right or wrong or fancy or sleep experiences or memories, and further every idea is accompanied by an emotional tone of pleasure or pain.

Control of these ideas is effected by practice and refusal to let them govern the emotions. Then super-mental contemplation (*samādhi*) becomes possible. If you are thinking of anything with dependence upon it, there is a motive of curiosity, or pleasure, or success, and though the thinking will help towards satisfaction you will still be in bondage. There is no harm in this, but the higher *samādhi*, without such motives, is best.

This higher outlook, which is understanding of consciousness can be reached towards by confidence in it, energy, memory, and the lower *samādhi*, or by devotion to God as free and self-existent Being, and to that universal Teacher, ever-present as *Om*.

There are many obstacles, such as disease, dullness, indecision, carelessness, worldliness, and wrong views, leading to distress, despair, nervousness, and disordered breathing, but the mind can be purified from all these by holding to this one truth.

Helps are increased sensitiveness, experiences of the peaceful inner light, thought of advanced beings who are free from desire, knowledge from dream or sleep, and meditation on your special interest.

Correct knowledge is seeing things as they are – seeing

1. This chapter is based on the *Yoga Sūtras* of Patanjali.

the known things, seeing the knowing, and seeing the knower. Beyond words and their meanings, knowledge, memory, opinions, comparisons, reasonings, lies the indefinable truth, to be attained by the higher contemplation (*samādhi*).

Yoga amid the affairs of daily life consists of strictness (for health, not indulgence, of the body), study of man (psychology, philosophy, religion), and devotion to God in all things, at all times.

These will reduce the great causes of trouble, which are ignorance, egotism, desires, aversions, and possessiveness. But meditation must be added to see their subtlety, and to eradicate them to the very root. Remember that future troubles are avoidable, and that they are due to the conjunction of the things with your consciousness. But you should in any given circumstances decide what you will do, feel, and think about, for you are consciousness only. Yet the world exists for the sake of the consciousness; you can make good use of every kind of experience.

There are eight things to practise in the process of yoga, from the condition in which men are to the height of insight (*viveka*) – abstinence, observance, posture, breathing, sense-control, concentration, meditation, and contemplation.

Abstinence is abstention from injury, untruth, theft, sensuality, and greed – or at least from enjoyment of these things.

Observance is attention to cleanliness, contentment, and the three already described as strictness, study of man, and devotion to God. All these ten lead also to the greatest prosperity of material and social living, as well as happiness of emotional, mental, and ethical living. They also conduce to the attainment of *samādhi*.

Posture should always be steady and pleasurable, never stiff and effortful, and should not be tensed from the mind.

Regulation of breath should be done for the sake of a good habit of breath – lengthy or slow, and fine, not rough.

Control of the senses should be practised so that they will

observe orders to abstain from attention or to pay attention according to your will.

*

Concentration is the holding of the mind to one object of attention, be it simple or complex, small or large, concrete, or abstract. Practice is according to ability – in most cases simple, small, and concrete in the beginning.

Meditation is full exercise of thought about that object.

Contemplation takes place when the thought-supply is exhausted, and one continues attentively looking, without desire or thought or wish or will, until intuition or insight or illumination comes.

These three are practised as one act, called *sanyama*, which leads to the reduction of the habit of mind-spreading and increase of the power of one-pointedness.

Sanyama is then a definite tool of mind, which can be used for gaining knowledge of various kinds, such as the understanding of sounds, and past and future, and what others have in their minds. Also for the acquisition of qualities, such as strength. Also for the development of deeper insight in connexion with hearing, feeling, seeing, tasting, and smelling; that is, clairvoyance. But these powers of the out-going mind are injurious to the higher contemplation. Specially mentioned are levitation, radiance, travelling in the ether, and control over various forms of matter.

From *sanyama* on the body will come correct form, beauty, strength, and compactness. On the senses, better functioning, character, and usefulness, leading on to great mental swiftness and penetrativeness.

But it is best of all when one realizes the absolute distinction between even the purest mind and the real man. Then indeed there is knowledge and mastery. Then when one is not coloured or bound even by that, there will indeed be Freedom, Independence.

Let those who are nearing this beware of pride, and of invitations from and to high estates. Discriminate, discriminate always, and among all things. Then, when the pure mind has become as pure as the real man, there will be Independence, even here.

*

In the fourth part of Patanjali's *Sūtras*, to which we now come, he gives the greater part of his explanation to the relation between mind and the world. He begins by saying that superior powers (*siddhis*) are in some cases congenital – men are born with them as a result of what they have done in previous lives. In some cases they are the result of taking certain drugs. In other cases they come from incantations (*mantras*) – the repetition of certain words or phrases. In other cases they arise from strict regimens (*tapas*). And, fifthly, they may also come about through contemplation (*samādhi*).

Changes from one condition or state to another come about through the flow of Nature, as when an agriculturist blocks or opens the channels for water to flow to selected patches of ground. 'Remove the obstacles and the results will appear' is a formula that applies to familiar material occurrences, to psychic powers, and also to spiritual realization. So it would seem that the exercises of yoga are not toilful manufacturing processes, but are in the main purifications, the getting rid of errors and bad habits.

There are artificial minds, which arise from egotism (*asmitā*), or personal reasons, and these presumably result from *samādhi* on the topics involved. Thus, it is interpreted, an advanced person can inspire several bodies at once, but the minds in those bodies will be subordinate to the chief one, and will have the limited scope of their originating intention. This reminds us of the idea that minds, like bodies, are temporary and that their contents acquired during life are emptied by assimilation or digestion into the spiritual substance or character of the real man beween death and the next incarnation. Or rather, as stated before, the relation is that between a little girl and her doll, in which the reflections in the mind even when the doll is absent play a greater part than the doll or the organs of sense and action in seeing and handling it.

A mind (*chitta*) thus produced by meditation differs from those produced by birth in that it has no separate container of karmic effects. As it is produced by an advanced yogi, the object of the extra mind is usually only to give wider response to the results of old karmas (actions), or to obtain some special kind of experience which he feels that he lacks.

The actions of such a yogi are neither black nor white (bad or good), but are concerned with those residues (*vāsanās*) from the past, or latent conditions of mind which are suitable for ripening. In general, it may be inferred, the theory is that karmas from the past, ripening in specific circumstances of life at the present time, are appropriate, on account of some sort of magnetic affinity, to the conditions of mind (*vāsanās*) also resulting from past thinking or mental actions and it is in the meeting of the two that valuable experience arises. In the case under consideration the yogi operating more than one mind is concerned only with such meeting, and not with ordinary personal desires, the personal choices of 'black' or 'white'.

The latencies (*vāsanās*) in the mind remain in suspense until the appropriate occasion occurs, and the occasion (which is a result of past karma) also remains in suspense until the latency is ripe. Here there is a touch of the theory that the internal sub-conscious ferment of the contents of the mind (*chitta*) constitute a sort of ripening, as is seen in modern psychology in the benefit of dreams. In this connexion I would definitely say that irrational dreams have a healing tendency for the emotions, analogous to the healing tendency of the body which occurs when we relieve it of the pressure of our minds in the condition we call sleep.

The impressions in the mind (*vāsanās*), or latencies, are next spoken of as having no beginning, but being a continuous succession of causes and effects in which, it is plainly stated, the will to live, or hope (*āshis*) is the constant support or basis or ground. No one is more practical than a *rāja-yogī*. He tells himself that he finds himself in the midst of something; he finds and accepts this simple fact. Then he asks himself not how it began but what is to be done about it. A person who has fallen into a pond does not then occupy himself with reflections as to how he fell in, but proceeds to the work of swimming. And yet at the back of his mind there is the philosophical thought that this will to accept the situation (the act of swimming) is part of his very consciousness, which is not of the same nature as the impressions in the mind (*vāsanās*), and can on no account be regarded as in the series. It we take the example of road and vehicle, this is the road, and the impressions are the vehicle going along it and constantly undergoing running repairs. Or in the example of a river. Who can say what a river is? Certainly one cannot define it as the water and the banks which are there, because these are constantly changing – coming and going. Similarly the will to be is not of the nature of the impressions.

This point of doctrine deserves the greatest emphasis and consideration. The impressions depend upon causes and effects, but these are not a simple line as ordinarily understood. It is not enough to say that the ink-bottle is on the table because someone put it there and the table is firm and stands on firm ground. It is there for a million reasons. The sun, the moon and stars, gravitation, chemical substance, and the rotation of the earth all played and play their parts. In fact the causality of anything being at any time where it is, is the convergence of all things. There is an absolutely enveloping causality. But this 'convergence of all things' is constant and not part of the series.

And yet further, as each thing is one factor in the convergence of influence upon all the others, we must declare it to be in possession of a share of the original causal power. In man, this will to live of which he is conscious is that very original power, and self-realization (*swasamvedana*) is the discovery of it. This is also independence (*kaivalya*) which the yogi attains at the time of his perfectly clear and one-pointed discrimination (*viveka*) of the distinction between the real man (*purusha, drashtri*) and all the clothing, trappings, and toys of mind and body.

In this highly theoretical part of Patanjali's account of

yoga, he goes so far as to say next that even the idea of time is to be transcended. He does not talk of 'the past', but 'what has gone', nor of the future, but of 'what is coming', and says that these have an existence 'of their own kind'. If causality is absolute, impregnable, inviolable, then we must infer that what is still to come has just as much pull as what has gone has push. So if we transfer this idea to the will to be, we can say that our will to be contains not only the impulse to live (which ignorance converts into desire) and to increase or enhance the living (the impulse to adventure) but also the will to fulfilment (*apavarga*). As a Western religious hymnist put it, 'Man will never rest until he finds his rest in Thee.'

As his next point, Patanjali warns us not to imagine that the things of the external world are unreal just because they are undergoing changes. He maintains that they are real or things-in-themselves (*tattwa*). His argument here is simple: first he says that any object is seen differently by different minds, and secondly that an object is not seen if it isn't there, or, in his words, the mind needs to be tinted by it. This has nothing to do – of course – with how the object came to be there. It may be the shape of a cloud due to various atmospheric causes, or it may be a table shaped by the hands of a carpenter directed by his thought. Still it affects the mind – the inner instrument – where the 'looker' sees it. In modern terms this is the theory of 'objective ideation'; ideation produces the form, but all the same that form, when produced, is independently objective. Patanjali states that even if an object were dependent upon one mind – that which produced it – it would not cease to exist when at some time that mind ceased to cognize it.

A subtly-observed reference to the real man (*purusha*), also called lord (*prabhu*), is here brought in. It is stated that the pictures or ideas in the mind are known to the real man only because he is not modified by them. The distinction may be brought out by considering a thermometer put into warm water. The mercury absorbs some of the heat. It is not correct to say that it indicates the heat of the water exactly, because it has cooled the water a little – though the expression is near enough for practical purposes. The case of the real man is, however, not like this. The real man is held to be a pure looker-on, entirely unaffected. It is only on that account that he can see truly. Any other sort of seeing would affect the thing seen. Then the seeing of it, so affected, would be wrong.

Shakarāchārya presents the same idea very clearly in his poem *Knowledge of the Self* (*Ātmabodha*), verse 52: 'The sage, though living among limitations, is unaffected by their qualities, like space.' Space has none of the qualities of the things 'in it', and so is unaffected by those things, space is, in fact, just nothing at all.

At the back of this view is the statement, constantly found in the deepest classical philosophy of India, that there is absolutely no relation between the spirit, or God, and the world. The proposition is really simple. The very conception of relationship belongs to the mind. It works by making comparisons, classifying and observing lines of causality, which are classifications in time-events. But what is beyond the mind is beyond all relativity. It is therefore unrelated, unaffected. But care must be taken here, for we must not dare to say that the unlimited cannot limit itself. If we say that the unlimited cannot at the same time be the limited, we should thereby be denying its unlimitedness. Therefore, let it be a mystery, as far as the mind is concerned. Still, not something unknowable to man, because he is not limited to mind. So, the real man is the witness, but not the doer with any conceivable sort of doing.

Conversely – Patanjali's next point – the mind is not self-illuminate. This means that we are conscious of the mind, but the mind itself is entirely unconscious. In evaluating this discovery – that the mind is unconscious – we have to avoid another possible error. It must not be assumed that the real man is the subject, and mind and body and world are the object. Subject and object are relative, and are classifications. Therefore it is that the mind is the subject and body plus world the 'object'. What occurred in observing the meditation was the discovery of the objectivity of the subject as well as the object in the subject-object relation. So we must not attach to the 'witness' (*sāk-shātkāra*) the conception of subject, even if we do allow ourselves to lump mind and matter together.

What we are doing in such a case is to find a *summum genus* or a top category which is beyond category. Compare it with our argument on the subject of reality. We said: 'The two highest categories of the known are 'something' and 'nothing'. Thus we may talk of things and of emptiness or absence or space, and then ask, 'What is it that the something and nothing have in common?' and answer 'Reality – they are both facts. So reality includes both something and nothing. We could not get on without having some nothing as well as some something always. Indeed, every observation or thought of ours uses both, for in looking at one thing we exclude others, and in giving definition to anything we perform exclusion as well as inclusion.' In comparing this with the ideas of subject and object we ask, 'What is it that these two have in common?' and shall have to reply, 'Consciousness', taking care to notice that when regarding subject we think of object while excluding it and when we speak of object we think of subject while excluding it.

Therefore the practical teachers tell their students who are about to go into meditation (*dhyāna*) and contemplation (*samādhi*) for self-realization, not to carry any of their preconceptions with them. This process is in another way akin to the religious study of God. 'Do not anthropomorphize God,' say the careful thinkers. 'Do not ascribe to God the qualities or actions of either mind or body.' Or, as the philosophers of old India would put it, do not confuse That (*Tat*) and This (*Idam*). God is not a great mind any more than a great body.

After stating his proposition that the mind is not self-illumined Patanjali continues his treatment of the same topic. He says that if when we see the mind as an object (as in the case when the student meditated on the flower) it is a case of one mind seeing another, a higher mind seeing a lower mind, as it were, there would need to be another still higher seeing that one, and so on infinitely. But in fact that is not the case, the real man not having the nature of a mind, but being beyond both subject and object. Besides, the mind, not being self-illuminate, cannot be the perceiver of another mind. When the mind 'sees' an object, it is only the real man who is seeing, with the mind as an instrument (*karana*) only.

Thus it is that the mind, with its innumerable latencies or tendencies, does not exist for its own enjoyment (being unconscious, as has been explained), but exists – in Patanjali's phrase – 'for the sake of another', that other being the real, man (*purusha*). The position may again be illustrated by the doll and the child, and extended to all things: the doll does not exist for its own enjoyment, but the sake of another, the child; further, the child's mind does not exist for its own enjoyment, but for the sake of the real man.

All the same – and here is a very subtle thought, requiring the greatest care in handling – the mind being coloured by both 'the looker' (*drashtri*; the same as the *purusha*) and 'the seen' (*drishya*) has everything within its scope – which, of course, includes the looker. This seems strange at first sight, does it not? For it seems as if we have promoted the mind to be the looker, quite in contradiction to what has just been said. The fact is, however, that the mind is never a looker. Only the looker is a looker, even when it uses the mind as its instrument to look at itself, not being in that supreme state in which the looker has transcended the mind and is knowing itself direct, not through any instrument.

This business of looking at the looker with the mind is exactly what we have been doing in the last few pages of this book. We cannot do better than that with the instrument of thought. It is again the case of a child knowing itself with the aid of a doll, the child being the only knower in the transaction; but here the doll is a mind-doll.

Some day there will be a transition from knowing the doll to knowing the knower of the doll, though in both cases there is only one knower – the doll never knows and the mind never knows. That transition, or rather awakening, is something different. When it comes, the mind becomes silent, quiet. It is not suprising that some have called it a new birth, a new beginning, an initiation in the proper sense of the word – in no sense negative or received from or through another, but 'from within'.

How then does this mind work for another? Patanjali puts it in the simple phrase: 'By combination' or 'By association' – with the real man, of course, as every tool or instrument does. Never can there be the liberating self-knowledge 'from within' if the mind and the operations of its latencies are mistaken for the within. It is not a mirror bright – it is only a doll. Yet not by clubbing it to death, that is by suppressing it, will the truth be seen. That will come about as the result of *samādhi* on the supreme distinction (*viveka*) or discrimination between the mind and the real man. The self is 'wonderful' (*āshcharyavat*), says the *Bhagavad Gītā*:

Someone sees this (body-owner) as wonderful; similarly another speaks (of this) as wonderful, and another hears of this as wonderful. Still although having heard about this, nobody knows.[1]

What an amount of philosophy there is here – in this word wonderful. Wonder is, then, above reason. All this reminds one of the statement: 'No man hath seen God at any time', with its emphasis upon the word man, the thinker, and the idea that one must be born again, even to the spirit.

Then there will be an end to the false idea of oneself – the *māyāvic* (illusory) *ahankāra* (I-maker). As Patanjali puts it:

On the part of him who sees the distinction (between mind and the real man), there is a turning away from thoughts about the nature of self.

Then the mind is deep in Discrimination and mainly pointed to Independence.[2]

Perhaps we ran a little ahead just now in our talk about the great discrimination, and looked at the perfection of it, or thought of it in its perfect moments. Patanjali has, however, brought it back to earth with his words 'mainly pointed'. We are reminded that our *samādhi* may not be

1. *Bhagavad Gītā*, ii, 29.   2. *Yoga Sūtras*, iv, 25, 26.

perfect, but is only teetering on the edge. We are reminded that even this highest *samādhi* is not the attainment itself, but only that last or highest act of the mind in which it is poised in its highest flight, in which it knows its own inadequacy, and surrenders. We are reminded that here we are seeing a dawnlight and not the full sun, but oh what a marvel that dawnlight is, arising over a dark world and illumining every part of it! 'The mind becomes deep in discrimination (*viveka*) and mainly pointed to Independence (*kaivalya*)' but 'At intervals there are other thoughts, arising from old habit-moulds (*sanskāras*)'.[1]

And these interrupting thoughts, he adds, must be dealt with as, in the course of meditation, we dealt with the five sources of all our troubles (*kleshas*).

Then he further adds, in the case of one having no more *intellectual* interest in the matter, on account of the increased understanding of discrimination (*viveka-khyāti*), there comes about that last and highest *samādhi* which is called 'the cloud of rectitude', which brings to a complete end all the trouble-makers (*kleshas*) and the actions (*karmas*) to which they lead.

In the case of one having no interest of any kind even in intellection, on account of Discrimination-knowledge, there is the Contemplation called 'cloud of rectitude'.

From that follows the retirement of Sources of Trouble and *karmas*.[2]

A few comments on the 'cloud of rectitude' may be in place. A rain-cloud in India is welcomed with great joy. From it come the refreshing and fertilizing waters, all good, very fundamental. So is the coming of virtue and all right conduct (*dharma*) when the trouble-makers (ignorance, egotism, attachment, aversion, and possessiveness) are gone from the mind and from the bodily life.

And now, what is still to be known becomes very little, 'on account of the infiniteness of knowledge' which the yogi has when he has become free of all coverings and impurities.

1. *ibid.*, iv, 27.   2. *ibid.*, iv, 29, 30.

Infiniteness of knowledge – how are we to understand this? Surely not as an infinite superfluity of useless information about everything – all the wheel-tracks in the mud. It is non-finiteness of knowledge when we can extract the infinite wisdom from every occasion. Then all are seen to be the same, and quantity gives place to quality. The most common occurrences of every day offer all that is needed for the vision of divine splendour and for the attainment of spiritual perfection. And as with one violin you may learn to play all violins, and with one mother you may learn to love all mothers, so the little that there is in a human life is enough, and enough is enough. Just as one need not seek outside oneself for the light, so one need not seek outside one's own small personal existence for the greater, unlimited, opportunity. With this realization comes the final death of greed, of hating, of fanaticism, of self-satisfaction, and of stupidity.

And from that comes the end of the series of transformations in the field of Nature,[1] and what had to be done has been done.[2]

Kaivalya, independence, freedom, has been won. The pure power of consciousness (*chitishakti*) stands in its own state (*swarūpa*).

1. Combinations of qualities of Nature – *tamas*, *rajas*, and *sattwa*.
2. *Yoga Sūtras*, iv, 32.

GLOSSARY OF SANSKRIT WORDS USED
IN THIS BOOK

Abhinivesa. Possessiveness, implying psychological dependency. Often applied especially to holding on to the body.

abhyāsa. Persevering practice (of yoga).

adharma. Breach of duty.

adhibhūta. The principle of extrinsic or objective existence.

adhidaiva. The principle of intrinsic or subjective existence.

adhikārī. Competent candidate.

adhiyajna. The principle of sacrifice, or the divine in manifestation, or Incarnation.

adhyāsa. Ascription to what is now seen of something seen before, as when a rope is mistaken for a serpent.

adhyātmā. The principle of self, which makes one conscious of self, quite apart from any definition or concept of self.

adrishta. The 'unseen'. A factor in all occurrences, including causative laws beyond the material, latencies or potentials not seen materially, such as the 'law of karma', and sometimes the actions of invisible entities.

adwaita. The non-dual; that 'than which there is no other'. Not one in the sense of an entity as distinguished from other entities.

aham. I.

ahankāra. 'The I-maker.' Often used to indicate the tendency to identify oneself with, or attribute to oneself, any of the features of the outside world, or of the body, or of the mind.

ahinsā. Non-injury, or harmlessness. The chief social virtue in yoga philosophy.

aishwarya. Desire for lordship or power, and therefore associated with pride. Fully understood psychologically, includes all desire to be pleased with oneself.

ajapā. Involuntary repetition; applied especially to the mantra or sound made in breathing, which is 'recited' 21,600 times every day, including night.

ājnā. A *chakra* or centre for certain functions, located at a level between the eyebrows.

ākāsha. Sky-matter; space; ether. The first of the material 'elements' or conditions of matter.

amrita. The nectar of immortality.

anāhata. A *chakra* or centre for certain functions, located at the level of the heart.

ānanda. Pure, unalloyed bliss or joy. Credited only to divine life.

anga. A 'limb' of yoga practice, of which there are eight.

antahkarana. The 'internal instrument' or organ. Refers to the entire mind, with all its functions.

antaranga. Inner limb (of yoga); the three practices of concentration, etc.
antarātman. Inner self.
apāna. One of the five vital airs, operating in the pelvic region, having downward movement.
aparigraha. Abstention from greed; the fifth of the moral abstinences.
ārāma. A pleasure-garden.
ardhanārīshwara. Shiva and his Shakti united in one form.
Arjuna. Disciple of Krishna, to whom the *Gītā* was spoken.
asamprajnāta. The superior kind of *samādhi*, in which the contemplation has no objective ground.
āsana. Seat; method of sitting; posture, for meditation or for health.
āshcharyavat. 'Wonderful', applied to the owner of the body.
ashwinī. One of the *mudrās*.
asmitā. 'I-am-ness'; egotism. One of the five *kleshas*, or causes of sorrow.
ātman or *ātmā.* The self, beyond mind and body.
āvarana. A veil or covering which hides or excludes part of the reality.
avatāra. A divine Incarnation, such as Krishna or Buddha.
avidyā. Ignorance, the chief of the five *kleshas* or sources of trouble.

Bandha. A muscular flexion which is 'held' for a little while; sometimes closing the exits, as at throat or anus.
basti or *vasti.* A method of cleaning the intestines.
bhadrāsana. The prosperity pose.
bhajana. A song of praise or hymn.
bhakti. Worship, religious devotion, devotion as service.
bhastrikā. A form of breathing rapidly, like bellows.
bhāvana. The dwelling of the mind's attention on some thing or idea.
bheda. A split; separation; division.
bhoga. Enjoyment, especially of the senses.
bhrāmarī. A breathing practice, connected with sound.
bhujungāsana. The cobra posture.
bhūmi. A ground; object of meditation.
bhūr-loka. The earth region.
bhūta. An element or state of matter, also popularly an entity, ghost, spook.
bhuvar-loka. The second region, above that of earth.
bīja. A seed; refers especially to a kind of contemplation, also to a kind of mantra. The *bīja* mantras are Laṁ, Vaṁ, Raṁ, Yaṁ, Haṁ and Oṁ.
bindu. A drop or point. Refers to the end part of mantric utterances ending in m.
bodhi. Supreme knowledge.
Brahma or *Brahman.* The utterly divine spirit, or God.
Brahmā. The third or working aspect of Brahma; creative deity.
brahmacharya. Conduct suitable for proceeding to God; especially control of sexual impulses.
Brahmadwāra. The door or gate of Brahman, where Kundalinī enters the spinal canal.

brāhmana. A man of the caste dedicated to the service of Brahman; also a certain portion of the Vedic scriptures, giving rules and explanations.

Buddha. The founder of Buddhism.

buddhi. The higher intelligence, concerned with not mere knowledge but wisdom; the faculty of valuing things for the advancement of life.

buddhi-yoga. The practice of *buddhi* or wisdom in the course of living.

Chakra. A 'wheel' or centre in the spine, governing a group of functions.

chit. Pure knowing, beyond the division of subject and object.

chitishakti. The power of knowing the chit.

chitrinī. A finer cord, stated to exist within the spinal cord.

chitta. The ordinary, more or less automatic mind; the lower mind, memory, etc.; the fourth function of mind as *antahkarana*, in Vedanta psychology.

Dākinī. The 'goddess' in the basic lotus.

dama. Control of the body and senses, especially in Vedanta practice.

dāna. Giving.

darbha. A sweet-smelling dried grass.

darshana. One of the six philosophical systems, or 'views'; sight of or visit to someone great.

dehī or *dehin.* The owner of the body; the self.

deva. A god or divine being.

devatā. A form of divinity, or a divine being having subordinate function.

devī. A goddess; a respectful term of address to ladies.

dhanurāsana. The bow posture.

dhāranā. Concentration, in the sense of continued or exclusive attention to one object or idea for a time.

dharma. The law; fundamental support; proper way of life; also duty.

dhīratā. Strength.

dhwani. A resonant sound.

dhyāna. Meditation. Continuity of mental process on one object or idea without leaving it.

dīrgha. Long.

drashtā or *drashtri.* The looker. The consciousness, which knows what is going on.

dridhatā. Strength.

dwesha. Dislike; hatred; antagonism.

Ekāgra. One-pointed.

Gate. First word of a certain Buddhist mantra.

Gautama. The founder of the Nyāya philosophy.

Gautama Buddha. The founder of Buddhism.

Gāyatrī. A famous and very sacred mantra, formerly recited only by brahmanas.

ghata. A pot or vessel, referring to the body.

ghī. Butter clarified by simmering, which makes it 'keep'.

gomukhāsana. The cow-faced posture.

granthi. A 'knot', or place in the *chitrini* where the ascending force meets with an obstruction to be pierced; analogous to the knots on a bamboo stem.

guna. A quality, especially one of the three inherent characteristics of *prakriti*, the basic substance of all things.

guru. A spiritual teacher – the word meaning weighty.

Hākinī. The 'goddess' in the eyebrow lotus.

hansa. A swan; title for a person in the third stage on 'the path' of spiritual advancement.

hare. First word of the mantra of sixteen names.

Hari. A name of Vishnu.

hatha-yoga. A school of yoga, dealing more especially with the bodily practices beneficial to an aspirant.

Ichchhā. The will, or a desire set or fixed by the will, also the basic function of mind.

idā. The left-side channel outside the spine.

idam. 'This'; all this, as distinguished from 'That' or what is beyond.

indriya. An organ of sense or action.

Īsha. A form of Shiva.

ishta-devatā. The *devatā* whose blessing or help an aspirant may desire.

īshwara-pranidhāna. Attentiveness to God.

Jālandhara. A *bandha* at the throat.

janma. Birth, incarnation.

japa. Repetition, especially of mantras.

jāti. Condition and circumstances in life, to which one is born.

jīvātmā. The Self of an individual.

jnāna. Knowledge of all kinds; but especially spiritual knowledge.

jnānendriya. An organ of knowledge, such as the eyes.

jyotis. An inner light.

Kaivalya. Spiritual independence.

Kākinī. The 'goddess' in the heart lotus.

kali-yuga. The current era of the world, difficult and full of strife, now more than 5,000 years old.

kāma. Desire for material pleasures.

kapāla bhāti. 'Cleansing the skull.'

karma. Doing, or work; action.

karmaphala. The fruit or result of action.

karma-yoga. Actions performed unselfishly, for the welfare of others.

karmendriya. An action-organ, such as the hands.

kathantā. Howness.

kaustubha. A jewel worn by Vishnu.

khecharī. A form of *mudra*, in which the tongue is inserted in the upper cavity.

khyāti. A field or outlook of knowledge.

kleshas. The five sources of trouble, of which ignorance is the chief.

klīm. A mantra.

koshas. Sheaths or bodies.

Krishna. The avatāra who spoke the *Gītā.*

kriyā. An action. Name given to the last three *niyamas*, as duties for every-day life. Action of Brahmā, which is thought.

kukkutāsana. The cock posture.

kumbhaka. The retention of breath.

kunda. The starting-place of *Kundalinī.*

Kundalinī. Vital 'electric' force or power residing near the base of the spine.

kūtastha. Established at the top; what stands above and beyond illusion.

kutīchaka. The 'hut-builder', second stage on 'the path'.

Lāghava. Lightness.

Lākinī. The 'goddess' in the navel lotus.

laulikī. Loosening the abdominal contents.

laya-yoga. Yoga by the use of the latent or sleeping power of *Kundalinī.*

loka. A world or region; a habitat.

Mahābandha. One of the principal *mudrās.*

Mahādeva. The great god; Shiva.

mahāvedha. A further development of the mahābandha.

manana. Thinking carefully and long.

manas. The mental faculty of comparing, classifying, reasoning, etc.

mandala. A magic circle or design.

mani. A jewel.

manipūraka. One of the *chakras*, at the level of the navel.

mantra. A word or sentence having some influence when recited with meaning.

mantrakāra. One competent to arrange a mantra.

mārga. A road, path, or way to the intended spiritual goal.

matsyāsana. The fish posture.

matsyendrāsana. The posture of the sage Matsyendra.

māyā. 'Illusion', not delusion. The world is an illusion, because seen as something which it is not, partly by veiling (*āvarana*) and partly by ascription (*adhyāsa*).

mayūrāsana. The peacock posture.

moksha. Liberation from the wheel of births and deaths.

mudrās. Various physical exercises aiming at some accomplishment or attainment of success, not concerned with the limbs as much as the *āsanas* are. They include the bandhas.

muktāsana. The liberated pose.

mukti. Liberation from the wheel of births and deaths.

mūlādhāra. The basic *chakra*, at the lower end of the spine.

mūla-shodhanā. Cleansing of the rectum.

mūrchā. Mind-fainting.

Nāda. Sound, especially the inner sound; also the prolongation of the sound in mantras such as Om.

nādī or *nādi.* A channel, corresponding somewhat to the modern idea of nerves.

namah. A salute.

Nārāyana. The god Vishnu; the supporter of life; the life of all lives.

nauli. An abdominal exercise, forming a ridge of muscle.

neti. 'Not this' or, more accurately, 'not so'. An expression used to warn the seeker of the divine or Brahman against anthropomorphic ascription, of the nature of body or mind.

neti-yoga. Nostril cleaning.

nididhyāsana. Meditation and contemplation.

nilimpa. A 'pictured' one, i.e. a god, thereby understood as pictured, but not as represented.

nirlipta. Unstainedness.

nirodha. Control, as control of ideas in the mind.

nirvāna. Extinction of all relation to the phenomenal world for a jivatma, resulting from extinction of all desire for it.

nirvichāra. Non-investigational (meditation).

nirvitarka. Non-inspectional (meditation).

niyamas. Observances of conduct or character, of which there are five.

Om. A mantric syllable indicating the supreme or rather sublime principle, or Brahman.

Padma. A lotus; another name for the *chakras.*

padmāsana. The lotus posture.

para. Beyond; used as a noun in the *Gītā* to indicate the supreme goal of life.

parā. Feminine of *para*; indicating the divine condition of *vāch.*

paramahansa. Title of a person on the fourth stage of the 'path'.

paramātmā. The supreme or sublime Self.

parivrājaka. 'Wanderer.' Title of a person on the first stage of the 'path'.

pashchimottanāsana. The drawing-back posture.

Patanjali. Author of the *Yoga Sūtras.*

pingalā. The channel on the right-hand side of the body, outside the spine.

prakāsha. Clearness, shiningness.

prakriti. The basic substance or principle of the entire phenomenal or manifest world.

pralaya. The state of periodic dematerialization or latency of the world.

prāna. The first of the five vital airs, operating in the region of the heart and lungs; a generic name for all five; breath.

pranava. Om.

prānāyāma. The practice of ordered breathing.

pranidhāna. Bowing before or glad yielding to *ishwara*, in delighted devotion to the divine when its presence is realized.

prāpta. What comes to us, which is not the result of present or recent efforts.

pratītya-samutpāda. Buddha's formula of the causal law of production as 'dependent origination'.

pratyāhāra. Withdrawal or control of the senses.

punarjanman. Birth again and again; rebirth.

pūraka. Drawing-in the air, inbreathing.

Purānas. Books of old legends regarding the creation of the world, etc.

pūrnāvatāra. The full *avatāra*; Krishna.

purusha. The spirit, entirely different from the prakriti.

Rajas. Energy, force, activity, restlessness – one of the three gunas of prakriti.

rāja-yoga. The yoga of kingship or mastery over the rāja mind.

rākinī. The 'goddess' in the pelvic lotus.

Rāma. A heroic and virtuous king, who was an avatāra.

rambhā. Plantain.

rechaka. Outbreathing.

Rudra. A form of Shiva.

rūpa. Form or body.

Sadāshiva. A form of Shiva.

sah. He or That.

sahaja. Dharma or karma to which one is born.

sahasrāra. The thousand-petalled lotus at the top of the head.

sākshātkāra. The spirit as witness having direct perception.

samādhāna. Steadiness in the pursuit of the accomplishments of 'the path'.

samādhi. Contemplation, the fulfilment of meditation.

samāna. One of the five vital airs, operating in the region of the navel.

samatwa. Evenness of outlook and reception, as regards all things and occurrences; equipoise.

samprajnāta. The kind of *samādhi* which has an objective *bhūmi*.

sanjnā also *sanna.* Perception or recognition responding to an object or idea.

sānkhya. The very old 'scientific' philosophy of India, which classifies all the contents of the known.

sansāra. The round of births and deaths; or reincarnations.

sanskāras. Mental impressions which, remaining unnoticed in the mind, set up impulses and trains of thought.

santosha. Contentment; pleasedness.

sanyama. The mind-poise which proceeds through concentration and meditation to contemplation (*samādhi*).

sāra. Essence.

sarvāngāsana. The pose of all the limbs.

sat. Reality; a character of the supreme, or Brahman.

sattwa. Orderliness, as one of the three *gunas* of *prakriti*; intelligence.

savichāra. Investigational (meditation).

savitarka. Inspectional (meditation).

shabda. Sound or word: the materially creative principle.

shabda-Brahman. Brahmā.

Shākinī. The 'goddess' in the throat lotus.

shakti. Power or ability; the feminine aspects or partners of the three great devas.

shaktichalanī. One of the *mudrās.*

shalabhāsana. The locust posture.

shama. Calming or controlling the mind.

shāmbhavī mudrā. The exercise named after Shambhu (Shiva).

Shankarāchārya. A famous philosopher who expounded and spread the advaita-vedanta outlook.

shāntih. Peace.

sharīra. A body, of which three are described – the dense, the subtle, and the causal.

shaucha. Cleanliness, of body and mind.

shavāsana. The corpse posture, giving maximum relaxation.

shesha. A name of the 'serpent of eternity', time.

shīrshāsana. The head-stand posture.

shishya. A pupil of a *guru.*

Shiva. The first or 'willing' aspect of Brahman, called the destroyer, as being concerned with regeneration and the goal of life.

shodanā. Purification, of six kinds.

shraddhā. Faith, sustained through progressive experience, and through intuition.

shravana. Hearing or listening to the doctrines, preparatory to thinking and meditating on them.

shrī. A polite form of address; Mr; also a name of Shiva's wife.

shrīmatī. A polite form of address; Mrs or Miss.

shrivatsa. A symbolic curl on the breast of Vishnu.

shuddha. Pure, clean.

siddhāsana. The adept's posture.

siddhi. An accomplishment; success; one of the eight occult powers.

sinhāsana. The lion pose.

skandhas. The five sensorial groups of Buddhism which go on changing from life to life.

sthiratā. Steadiness.

sthūla-sharīra. The dense body.

sukha. Pleasure, happiness.

sukhāsana. The 'comfortable' posture.

sūkshma-sharīra. The subtle body.

sushumnā. The spinal cord.

sūtras. Condensed statements strung together to give an outline of a philosophy, such as the *Yoga Sūtras* of Patanjali.

swādhishthāna. One of the *chakras*, at the level of the generative organs.

swādhyāya. Study of oneself, or of one's own scriptures or school of philosophy, or in general of what it means to be a man.

swāhā. The terminal word of some mantras.

swar-loka. The third region of the world, beyond *bhuvar-loka*, generally identified with *swarga* or heaven.

swāra-sādhaka. Breath-practiser.

swarga. Heaven.

swarūpa. One's own true form or nature.

swasamvedana. The understanding of oneself.

swastika. An auspicious sign, the equal-armed cross with bent ends suggesting rotating or the cross in activity.

swastikāsana. The 'auspicious' seat.

Tamas. Darkness, inertia; one of the three *gunas* of *prakriti*.

tanmātras. The five senses as such; the essence of sound, sight, etc.

tantras. Certain scriptures in the form of a dialogue between Shiva and his Shakti, forming a set of rules for ritual, worship, discipline, meditation, and the attainment of powers.

tapas. Austerity, often exaggerated into self-mortification, but in yoga, body-conditioning for the removal of impurities and the perfection of the body and the senses.

tāra. Crossing over.

tārasāra mantra. The '*Om namo Nārāyanāya*'.

tat. 'That'; the Beyond, other than 'this'; Brahman.

tattwa. 'Thatness'; the truth about something, or thing-in-itself.

trātaka. A *hatha-yoga* exercise for the eyes.

trikona. A triangle.

trimūrti. The three great gods.

Udāna. One of the five vital airs, operating upwards from the throat.

uddīyāna. An exercise of the abdominal muscles.

Umā. A name of Shiva's wife.

Upanishads. The philosophical sections of the Vedas.

vairāgya. 'Uncolouredness'; not being incited to desire by external objects.

vajra. A thunderbolt; a diamond; something strong, hard, irresistible; one of the spinal channels.

vajrāsana. The adamantine posture.

vajrolī. 'Thunderbolt' exercise.

vāmaprakāsha. Lovely shiningness, a description of *dhyāna*.

vasti. Internal cleansing.

vāyus. The vital airs in the body.

Vedanā. Residual impulses latent in the mind; feelings and sensations.

vedānta. The end or high point or ultimate philosophy of the Vedas.

Vedas. The ancient scriptures of India.

vibhūtis. Examples of divine power or expression.

vichāra. Serious and continued thought.

vijnāna (vinnana). Cognition of the objective world.

vikalpa. Imagination; fancy; planning.

vikshepa. 'Throwing-out'; creation by mind, according to limited and incomplete understanding.

vipākas. Results of karmas, when they react upon the doer.

viparītakaranī. The inverted exercise.

virāsana. The hero posture.

vishesha. Especial, particular.

Vishnu. The second of the three aspects of Brahman; the preserver of life.

vishuddha. The *chakra* at the level of the throat.

vitarka. Inspection or discernment.

viveka. Discrimination, especially between the real and the limited.

vrikshāsana. The tree pose.

vritti. A whirlpool; in the flow of mind, an idea.

vyāna. The vital air which operates all over the body.

Yajna. A sacrifice; the principle of sacrifice or mutual maintenance.

Yajnavalkya. A great sage, in the Upanishads.

yama. The five moral abstinences.

yantra. A design used in magic or in meditation.

yoga. 'Union'; the method and practice leading to conscious union of the human being with the divine principle.

yogārūdha. 'Mounted on yoga.' Well established in yoga practice.

yogī or *yogin.* One who practises yoga.

yoginī. A female yogī.

yukta. Joined with or keeping to, as in buddhi-yukta.

Zen. A form of meditation or meditative outlook and attitude to life developed in Japan.

ORIGINAL SANSKRIT BOOKS AND TREATISES QUOTED

Aparokshānubhūti.
Atmanātma Viveka.
Bhagavad Gītā.
Chhāndogya Upanishad.
Dhyānabindu Upanishad.
Garuda Purāna.
Gheranda Sanhitā.
Gopālatāpani Upanishad.
Hathayoga Pradīpikā.
Kalisantārana Upanishad.
Kundalinī Yoga.
Krishna Upanishad.
Mahānirvāna Tantra.
Mahā-prajñā-pāramitā-hridaya.

Mandala Brāhmana Upanishad.
Nārāyana Upanishad.
Saundarya Laharī.
Shāndilya Upanishad.
Shatchakra Nirūpana.
Shiva Sanhitā.
Tārasāra Upanishad.
Trishikhi Brāhmana Upanishad.
Vedānta Sāra.
Viveka Chūdāmani.
Yoga Sūtras.
Yogakundalī Upanishad.
Yogatattwa Upanishad.

BOOKS ON YOGA IN ENGLISH

This bibliography is only a representative selection from the great volume of literature on the subject of yoga.

Aiyengar, Srinivasa. *Hatha-yoga Pradīpikā.* Bombay (Tukaram Tatya).
Arnold, C. H. *110 Years of Youth through Yoga.* London (L. N. Fowler).
Arnold, Sir Edwin. *The Song Celestial,* and *The Light of Asia.*
Atreya, B. L. *Self-Realization* (from the Yoga Vashistha). Benares (Indian Bookshop).
Aundh, the Raja of. *The Ten-point Way of Health.* London (Dent).
'Avalon, Arthur'. *See* Woodroffe, Sir John.
Bailey, Alice. *Light of the Soul* (trans. of *Yoga Sūtras* of Patanjali). New York (Lucis Press).
Bāla Sanyāsī. *Rāja-yoga with Nava Kalpa.* Bangalore (Parashakti Ashram).
Ballantyne & Shastri. *Yoga Sūtras of Patanjali.* Calcutta (Sushila Gupta).
Behanan, K. T. *Yoga, a Scientific Evaluation.* London (Macmillan).
Bernard, T. *Hatha Yoga.* New York (Columbia Univ. Press).
Besant & Das. *The Bhagavad Gītā* (with word analysis). Madras (Theosophical Publ. House).
Bose & Haldar. *Tantras, their Philosophy.* Calcutta (Oriental Publ. Co.).
Chatterjee, Mohini. *Crest Jewel of Wisdom.* Madras (Theosophical Publ. House).
Cohen, S. S. *Guru Ramana.* Madras (Vishwanatha).
Coster, G. *Yoga and Western Psychology.* London (Oxford Univ. Press).
Danielou, J. *Yoga, the Method of Reintegration.* New York (University Books).

Dasgupta, Surendranath. *The Study of Patanjali*. Calcutta (University).

Dasgupta, Surendranath. *Yoga as Philosophy and Religion*. London (Kegan Paul).

Day, H. *The Study & Practice of Yoga*. New York (University Books).

Desai, Mahadev. *The Gītā According to Gandhi*. Ahmedabad (Navajivan Publ. House).

Dwivedi, M. N. *The Yoga Sūtras of Patanjali*. Madras (Theosophical Publ. House).

Edgerton, Franklin. *The Bhagavad Gītā*. London (Oxford Univ. Press).

Evans-Wentz, W. Y. *Tibetan Book of the Great Liberation*. London (Oxford Univ. Press).

Evans-Wentz, W. Y. *Tibet's Great Yogī, Milarepa*. London (Oxford Univ. Press).

Goddard, Dwight. *A Buddhist Bible*. New York (Dutton).

Humphreys, Christmas. *Buddhism*. London (Penguin).

Indra Devi. *Forever Young, Forever Healthy*. Englewood Cliffs (Prentice-Hall).

Jha, Ganganatha. *The Yoga Darshana*. Bombay (Tukaram Tatya).

Jha, Ganganatha. *The Yogasāra Sangraha*. Bombay (Tukaram Tatya).

Lounsbery, G. C. *Buddhist Meditation in the Southern School*. London (Luzac).

Mādhavānanda, Swami. *Viveka Chudāmani*. Mayavati, Almora, India (Advaita Asram).

Mahādeva Shāstri. *Bhagavad Gītā* (with Shankara's Commentary). (Mysore).

Mitra, Rājendralal. *Yoga Aphorisms.*

Nārāyānanda, Swāmī. *Secrets of Mind-Control*. Rishikesh, India (Prasad).

Nārāyānanda, Swāmī. *The Primal Power in Man*. Rishikesh, India (Prasad).

Nārāyanaswāmī Aiyar. *Thirty Minor Upanishads*. Madras (Adyar).

Nikhilānanda, Swami. *The Bhagavad Gītā*. New York (Ramakrishna-Vivekananda Centre).

Prasād, Rāma. *Nature's Finer Forces*. Madras (Theosophical Publ. House).

Prasād, Rāma. *Aphorisms of Yoga, by Patanjali*. Allahabad (Pānini Office).

Premānanda, Swāmi. *Srimad Bhagavad Gītā*. Boston (Christopher Publ. House).

Radhakrishnan, S. *The Principal Upanishads*. London (Allen and Unwin.)

Radhakrishnan, S. *The Bhagavad Gītā*. London (Allen and Unwin).

Radhakrishnan & Moore (editors). *Source Book of Indian Philosophy*. Princeton, N.J. (Princeton University Press).

Rele, Vasant G. *The Mysterious Kundalinī*. Bombay (D. P. Taraporevala).

Sadamanda, Swami. *Vedānta Sāra.*

Sarma, D. S. *The Bhagavad Gītā*. Triplicane, Madras (Current Thought Press).

Shankarāchārya. *Compendium of Rāja Yoga Philosophy*, containing: *Aparokshānubhūti, Atmanātma Viveka, Shrī Vākya Sudhā, Crest Jewel of Wisdom*. Adyar, Madras (Theosophical Publ. House).

Shāstri, Hari Prasad. *Yoga*. London (Foyle).

Shivānanda, Swāmī. *Kundalinī Yoga*. Rishikesh, India (Divine Life Society).

Shivānanda & Vishnudevānanda. *Practical Guide for Students of Yoga*. Hong Kong (Divine Life Society).

Spiegelberg, F. *Spiritual Practices of India*. San Francisco (Greenwood Press).

Subba Row. *Esoteric Writings*. Bombay (Rajaram Tukaram).

Sukul, D. R. *Yoga and Self-culture*. New York (Yoga Institute of America).

Tookārām Tātya. *The Bhagavad Gītā*. Bombay (Tattvavivechaka Press).

Venkataraman, S. *Select Works of Shankarāchārya*. Madras (Natesan).

Vidyāranya, Srish Chandra. *Gheranda Sanhitā*. Adyar, Madras (Theosophical Publ. House).

Vidyāranya, Srish Chandra. *Daily Practice of the Hindus*. Allahabad (Pānini Office).

Vivekānanda, Swami. *Raja Yoga*. New York (Ramakrishna-Vivekananda Centre).

Wood, Ernest. *Practical Yoga: Ancient and Modern* (with trans. of *Yoga Sūtras*). London (Rider) and New York (Dutton).

Wood, Ernest. *The Glorious Presence* (with trans. of *Dakshināmūrti Stotra*). London (Rider) and New York (Dutton).

Wood, Ernest. *The Dancing Shiva* (with trans. of *Shiva Tāndava Stotra*). Madras (Ganesh).

Wood, Ernest. *The Bhagavad Gītā Explained* (with trans.). Los Angeles (New Century Foundation).

Wood, Ernest. *Great Systems of Yoga*. New York (Philosophical Library).

Wood, Ernest. *Yoga Dictionary*. New York (Philosophical Library).

Wood, Ernest. *Garuda Purāna*. Allahabad (Pānini Office).

Wood, Ernest. *Occult Training of the Hindus*. Madras (Ganesh).

Wood, Ernest. *Mind and Memory Training*. New York (Occult Research Press).

Wood, Ernest. *Intuition of the Will*. Madras (Theosophical Publ. House).

Wood, Ernest. *Concentration, a Practical Course*. Madras (Theosophical Publ. House).

Woodroffe, Sir John. *The Garland of Letters*. Madras (Ganesh).

Woodroffe, Sir John. *Shakti and Shakta*. Madras (Ganesh).

Woodroffe, Sir John. *The Serpent Power*. Madras (Ganesh).

Woods, J. H. *Yoga-System of Patanjali*. Cambridge, Mass. (Harvard University Press).

Yesudian and Haich. *Yoga and Health*. New York (Harper).

INDEX

Abdominal uplift, 133

Abstention (*yama*), 37, 38, 45, 46, 178, 236

Acceptance, of people and things, 54, 55

Actions, 219, 220, 221, 222, 223, 227, 233, 239; 'entire', 227; 'fruit of', 223

Act of Inversion (*Viparītakaranī*), 115, 134, 135

Ājña Chakra. See Chakras (Brow centre)

Aloneness (*Kaivalya*), 19. *See also* Independence

Alphabet, Sanskrit, 150, 151

Amulets, 210

Ānanda (Joy), 71, 164, 187, 194

Ananta (endless time), 193

Angas. See Limbs of yoga

Annihilation, theory of, 21, 23

Antahkarana (inner instrument, or mind), 162

Antaranga. See Limbs of yoga

Antarātman (inner self), 174. *See also* Self

Anthropomorphism, 26, 243

Aparigraha. See Non-greed

Aphorisms. *See* Kapila; *Yoga Sūtras*

Ardhanārīshwara, 166, 168

Arjuna, disciple of Krishna, 75, 76, 205, 217, 225, 230, 233

Asamprajñāta. See Contemplation (non-cognitive)

Āsanas. See Exercises; Posture

Ashwinī-mudrā, 171

Asmitā (attainment), 71, 187

Ātmā (Supreme Self), 86, 112–113nn., 137, 167, 223, 227. *See also* Self

Atmanātma Viveka, 123n.

Attentiveness, observance of, 43, 44, 136, 188, 189, 230, 233; reward, 56, 57

Austerity, observance of, 41, 78; reward, 55, 56

Avatāra. See Incarnation

'Awakening', to yogic life, 14

Baradā Tantra, 206

Being. acts of, 72; primeval, 174

Beyond, the (*Para*), 27, 28, 30, 72, 124, 125, 195, 226

Bhadrāsana, 120. *See also* Posture (miscellaneous)

Bhagavad Gītā, 20, 25, 27, 28, 33, 34, 39, 40, 41, 42, 75, 76, 90, 112, 130, 169n., 191, 205n., 245, 216–34; allusions to the Beyond, 27; allusions to Nirvana, 25; definition of yoga, 216; methods of yoga, 216; 'looking between the eyebrows', 130; on the Self, 33, 34, 245; on posture, 112; survey of teaching of, 216–34

Bhajans (praises), 210

Bhaktı-yoga, 209, 210, 231

Bharadwaja. 201

Bhastrikā, 104, 105, 172

Bhrāmarī (Beetle exercise), 135, 137

Bhujangāsana, 118. *See also* Posture (recumbent)

Bhūmi (subject of thought), 183

Bhūr, 196

Bhuvah, 196

Bhuvaneshwar, temple, 190

Births, as place of pain, 229; method of, 51

Bodhidharma (Buddhist monk), 34

Body, the, as outer instrument, 38; 'brain' of, 178, 180; channels of, 174 ff.. 182; functions, 176, 178; means of perception, 77; powers, 55; physical practices for, 55; structure, 180, 181, 182; vital airs in relation to functions, 175;

INDEX